Barbara O'Neill Natural |

Remedies Lost Collection:

Over 800 Natural Remedies Inspired by Barbara's

Knowledge to Discover Holistic Health, Well-Being, and

a Toxic-Free Lifestyle

By

Serena Dolton

Table of Contents

2 Exclusive Bonus

Bonus 1: Access over 20 hours of exclusive videos from Dr. Barbara O'Neill

Bonus 2: Grow Your Own Food: A comprehensive guide to cultivating your own fruits, vegetables, and herbs at home.

BOOK 1:

Discovering Dr. Barbara O'Neill

Introduction to dr. Barbara O'Neill's philosophy

Natural healing, holistic wellbeing, and preventative care are at the center of the concept of well-known naturopaths and health educators.

Dr. Barbara O'Neill. The notion that, given the correct circumstances, the body has the innate capacity to cure itself is fundamental to her views. In her advocacy for a balanced lifestyle, Dr. O'Neill highlights the significance of detoxification, diet, and lifestyle management. She advocates for frequent bodily purification, a plant-based diet, and lifestyle modifications, including getting enough sleep, exercising, and managing stress. With a focus on empowering people to take charge of their own health, her holistic approach incorporates physical, emotional, and spiritual wellbeing.

Natural and traditional methods are the foundation of Dr. O'Neill's philosophy and often function as a substitute for or addition to orthodox treatment. She has encountered opposition and legal issues from the conventional medical profession, but her teachings have gained a sizable following among those looking for natural and preventative health remedies. Her emphasis on empowerment and education is to support people in adopting sustainable, holistic habits that improve overall wellbeing and in making educated choices about their health.

A number of fundamental ideas form the basis of Dr. Barbara O'Neill's philosophy and direct approach to wellness and health. These values reflect her faith in the efficacy of alternative therapies and the significance of a wholistic approach to wellness.

Natural healing

Dr. O'Neill's theory is based on the idea that the body is capable of self-healing. She suggests that exposure to chemicals, bad food, and improper living arrangements are the root causes of many contemporary health problems. She feels people may regain their health and stave off illness by going back to natural and holistic approaches.

Nutrition

Food, in Dr. O'Neill's opinion, really is medicine. She stresses that maintaining good health and preventing sickness starts with eating a balanced diet. Her dietary advice is centered on whole, plant-based meals that enhance general health and provide vital nutrients.

Detoxification

The foundation of Dr. O'Neill's ideology is detoxification. She thinks that a lot of health issues are mostly brought on by the buildup of toxins in the body. Consistent detoxification procedures are necessary to keep your health at its best.

Lifestyle changes

Dr. O'Neill stresses the need to modify one's lifestyle to support general wellbeing. These adjustments aim to establish a well-rounded, healthful lifestyle that promotes long-term wellbeing.

Holistic approach

Dr. O'Neill's concept of health is centered on a holistic approach. According to her, genuine health is all about being in good bodily, emotional, and spiritual health. Achieving good health requires addressing each of these factors.

Criticism and controversy

The method used by Dr. Barbara O'Neill has not been without criticism. She has drawn criticism for her ideas and practices, especially from the mainstream medical establishment.

Lack of scientific validation: according to her detractors, some of her tactics are not backed up by solid scientific data. They issue a warning that using just natural therapies might be risky, particularly in cases of severe illness that call for the use of conventional medical care.

Potential risks: there are worries that following her advice might cause people to skip essential medical care, which could be harmful. Before making big adjustments to their health routine, people should always speak with healthcare specialists.

Regulatory actions: among the regulatory obstacles Dr. O'Neill has had to overcome is an Australian restriction on his practicing naturopathy. Regulatory agencies questioned her credentials and the veracity of her advice, citing concerns for public safety.

Despite these obstacles, Dr. O'Neill and others who support her contend that many of her teachings are rooted in long-standing traditional traditions and that contemporary medicine often ignores the advantages of natural therapy.

Who is Dr. Barbara O'Neill?

Renowned Australian naturopath and health educator Dr. Barbara O'Neill is well-known for her support of holistic wellness and natural therapy.

Over the course of her multi-decade career, Dr. O'Neill has amassed a sizable following via her books, online material, seminars, and workshops. Her guiding principles stress the need for detoxification and lifestyle modifications, the body's inherent capacity for self-healing, and diet's vital role.

Early life and education

Early in childhood, Dr. Barbara O'Neill's interest in holistic therapy and her own experiences molded her path into the field of natural health and wellbeing. She was reared in an atmosphere that emphasized natural living and conventional therapeutic methods, having been born and raised in Australia. These early inspirations greatly impacted her eventual work as a health educator and naturopath.

A constant quest for knowledge in the areas of nutrition, alternative medicines, and naturopathy defined Barbara's educational career. She enrolled in formal education in order to combine academic knowledge with real-world applications and get a better grasp of natural health concepts. She received a wide and complete skill set from her studies, which includes significant study in holistic health practices, nutrition, and herbal medicine.

Professional career

Over the course of her many decades in the workforce, dr. O'Neill has had a significant influence on the natural health industry. Her dedication to promoting natural treatment techniques and teaching others is evident in her work. These are significant turning points and facets in her career:

Naturopathic practice

Initially, Dr. O'Neill worked as a licensed naturopath, using her training to assist people in achieving better health naturally. Her areas of expertise were natural medicines, customized food plans, and holistic health evaluations. Many of her customers connected with her belief that treating health problems at their core instead of just treating their symptoms was a good idea.

Health educator and speaker

Being a health educator and speaker is one of Dr. O'Neill's most important professional roles. She has shared her knowledge on a range of health-related issues by conducting seminars and workshops all around the world. Several topics have been addressed in these instructional seminars, such as:

Nutrition: the value of entire foods and a plant-based diet in preserving health.

Detoxification: methods for eliminating toxins from the body and enhancing general health.

Natural remedies: using plants, essential oils, and other elements of nature to promote well-being.

Holistic health: it refers to the integration of mental, emotional, and spiritual aspects of well-being for overall wellbeing.

Dr. O'Neill is in high demand as a speaker at medical conferences and public gatherings because of her engaging speaking style and aptitude for simplifying complicated health topics.

Author and content creator

Apart from giving speeches, dr. O'Neill is a published author of many books and a large number of papers on natural health. Her written works are intended to educate a wider readership about the fundamentals of natural healing and to provide helpful advice to those who want to become healthier. Her significant writings include books on nutrition, natural cures, and detoxification.

In order to reach a wider audience, dr. O'Neill has also embraced digital channels. She has been able to reach a worldwide audience via producing webinars, video lectures, and online courses. She keeps spreading her expertise and encouraging others to lead better lives via various platforms.

Health retreats and programs

Her career has also benefited greatly from the creation of wellness programs and health retreats. Under the direction of Dr. O'Neill and her staff, these retreats provide participants with an immersion experience in natural health techniques. Usually, the programs consist of:

Detoxification protocols: organized detox regimens help purify the body and restore wellness.

Nutritional guidance includes cooking classes and individualized diet programs to educate participants on how to make healthful meals.

Physical exercise: exercise programs designed to accommodate varying levels of fitness that highlight the significance of consistent physical exercise.

Stress management: methods to control stress and enhance mental health, such as yoga, meditation, and relaxation techniques.

These retreats provide a safe space where people may transform their health and personally feel the advantages of Dr. O'Neill's methodology.

Controversies and challenges

Throughout her career, Dr. Barbara O'Neill has faced criticism. Her focus on alternative medicine and mistrust of traditional medicine have drawn criticism from several regulatory agencies and medical experts. Principal issues of disagreement consist of the following:

Scientific validation: according to critics, there is insufficient scientific evidence to support certain of dr. O'Neill's procedures. They issue a warning that using natural therapies exclusively may be dangerous, especially in cases of severe illnesses that call for the use of conventional medical care.

Regulatory actions: Dr. O'Neill was subject to regulatory action in 2019 after being prohibited from practicing naturopathy by the new South Wales health care complaints commission (hccc). The hccc raised doubts over the efficacy and safety of her medical advice, especially with regard to major illnesses like diabetes and cancer.

Dr. O'Neill insists that her strategy is founded on a blend of conventional knowledge and modern ideas in spite of these difficulties. She and others who support her contend that traditional medicine often fails to recognize the advantages of natural remedies and that her teachings provide viable alternatives for anyone looking for holistic approaches to health.

Legacy and influence

The impact of Dr. Barbara O'Neill goes beyond her clinical work and teaching activities. A new generation of wellness lovers and health professionals who value natural and holistic approaches to wellbeing have been inspired by her. Her lessons inspired many others to take charge of their health, make wise decisions, and embrace long-term, sustainable routines that support wellbeing.

Dr. O'Neill has made a significant contribution to the area of natural health by reaching a worldwide audience via her publications, seminars, internet material, and one-on-one consultations. Those looking for alternative health treatments continue to be drawn to her dedication to empowering and educating others.

In the fields of naturopathy and natural health, Dr. Barbara O'Neill is well-known for her comprehensive approach and commitment to teaching others. Her upbringing, which was influenced by her own experiences and dedication to lifelong learning, has helped her succeed in her work as a naturopath, health educator, author, and speaker. Her idea of natural health, adequate nutrition, detoxification, and lifestyle modifications has gained a sizable following while encountering criticism and regulatory obstacles.

Dr. O'Neill has significantly influenced the area of natural health with her work, encouraging people to adopt holistic lifestyles and take charge of their health. Her commitment to empowering and educating people and her advocacy of a natural and preventative approach to health have left a lasting legacy that continues to impact many people worldwide.

BOOK 2:

Understanding Your Body's

Healing Power

Everyone knows how important listening skills are. Active listening fosters cooperation, trust, and the avoidance of misunderstandings. Still, how many of us pay attention to what our bodies are telling us? To enhance your health, learn about your body.

These are some possible messages from your body. You'll discover that you both speak the same language if you pay careful attention!

The organs and tissues that make up your body are intricate structures composed of many cells. Eleven organ systems—including the circulatory, skeletal, endocrine, digestive, and respiratory systems—are made up of these organs. All these systems work together to form the well-oiled machine that is your body; yet, if one of them has a problem, it may negatively impact your quality of life and cause problems with everyday functioning.

Being proactive with your health requires an understanding of your body, how it works, and how your surroundings affect the choices you make about your health. Although everybody works in much the same manner, differences in your DNA and the environment you live in may greatly influence your health.

A healthy philosophy starts with recognizing these elements and comprehending how they affect your health.

The body's innate ability to heal

The human body has an incredible, remarkable, and enduring ability to repair itself. Disease usually results from mistreating our bodies or depriving them of necessities for long-term health.

Your body is very capable of self-healing. Your body should respond to injuries or illnesses swiftly and effectively, healing itself back to full strength. Given the superior architecture of our bodies, why then do 20.4% of adult Americans experience chronic pain, and over 40% of Americans suffer from chronic diseases?

The limitations of what we now know contribute to the response. Some of the methods by which our bodies repair themselves are quite well understood and known to us; others are still likely to be unknown to science, and there may be other mechanisms that we haven't even begun to consider. Medical care and scientific research have spent many decades addressing symptoms, often with drugs or surgery. This method works well when you require antibiotics for a potentially fatal illness or to fix a fractured bone, but it falls short in other scenarios.

A healthy body fends off infections, mends injuries, eradicates cancerous cells, fixes damage, and slows down the aging process. But it takes more than just going to the doctor when anything goes wrong to maintain and restore health so your body can use its natural healing mechanisms.

How does your body heal itself?

There are several ways that healing occurs. This is a very basic synopsis of a handful of them.

When a cell becomes sick, it has the ability to repair itself by replicating to replace lost or damaged cells. Your body instantly starts to create new cells to repair the harm if you break a bone. Your blood clots around cut skin to halt bleeding, while white blood cells eliminate harmed or dead cells, and new, healthy cells heal the injured tissue. Additionally, daily wear and tear is immediately addressed. Our bodies are actually always repairing harm and forming new, healthy tissue.

Toxins, bacteria, and viruses are among the invaders that our immune system is designed to combat. Foreign objects are captured by mucus, organisms are killed by acids found in different organs, and invaders are consumed and destroyed by phagocytes, a kind of white blood cell. When a virus infiltrates one of our cells, natural killer cells detect and eliminate the contaminated cell. Although it may appear to be a problem, inflammation is really your body's response to an injury or infection, enabling your immune system to concentrate on healing the affected or infected area. Your body raises its temperature to eliminate bacteria and viruses when you have a fever. Additionally, the rise in body temperature sets off specific cellular processes that aid in the body's defense against the infection. Stem cells also help bodies repair and regenerate. Embryonic stem cells proliferate and differentiate into every cell type required for a child to grow into a fully formed human during its development inside the womb. The progeny of embryonic stem cells, known as adult stem cells, remain after the body has developed. When your adult stem cells divide, a healthy, mature cell of a certain type and identical daughter stem cells are produced. Every kind of adult stem cell, in contrast to embryonic stem cells, can only differentiate into a specific kind of tissue. For instance, neural stem cells aid in the regeneration of nerve tissue in the brain and spinal cord, epithelial stem cells renew skin, and mesenchymal stem cells have the capacity to regenerate bone, fat, muscle, and cartilage cells. Although adult stem cells have a long half-life, they are not immortal and will eventually cease to proliferate as effectively as they did when you were a child.

Why do our bodies fail to heal themselves?

Numerous things hamper the body's innate ability to mend itself. While some of these are readily apparent, others are yet unknown to us. We are aware that your body needs regular exercise, a nutritious diet, and enough restorative sleep. Toxins and stress of all kinds are harmful. Your mental state might also affect your health.

It's critical to get the recommended quantity and quality of sleep. You repair and regenerate much of your body when you sleep. In addition to reducing the length of time your body can recover itself, sleep deprivation impairs your immune system. Due to your increased susceptibility to disease, your body must focus its healing energies on curing the illness rather than healing injuries sustained from normal daily activities. A nutritious diet rich in nutrients is also essential for the healing process. Your body needs it for the best possible health and vigor. On the other hand, environmental pollutants can accumulate in your diet and cause significant harm to your entire system. In addition to causing inflammation, diet can aggravate digestive issues.

Even a short stroll can increase blood flow, which removes toxins from your body and supplies your cells with nutrition and oxygen. It lessens emotional tension and enhances your mentality and sleep quality. Studies indicate that physical activity not only enhances overall well-being but also may contribute to cancer and aging. How could that be true? Elite athletes had much longer telomeres than the general population, but sedentary lifestyles are associated with shorter telomeres. The protective structures known as telomeres are found at the ends of chromosomes and serve to shield DNA. When the telomere becomes sufficiently short, DNA is more susceptible to damage, which can lead to aging- or cancer-causing processes. Another significant contributor to ill health is free radicals. They are crucial in removing trash that has caused damage to the cell. On the other hand, free radical generation is elevated by infection, stress, and inflammation. Overproduction of free radicals by the body leads to oxidative stress, which ruins DNA and cells and results in disease.

When stem cells run out of energy and are unable to replicate and create new tissue, your body's ability to heal and regenerate is also compromised. While the exact causes of the decline in stem cell numbers and efficiency with age are yet unknown, oxidative stress, chronic illness, and telomere shortening are a few potential causes.

The healing power of nature

When a few Japanese researchers set out to see if spending time in nature has any unique, therapeutically curative effects, it seemed more like a joke than a scientific study. They were motivated by recent advice from the Japanese forest agency, which started encouraging people to go for walks in the woods for improved health in the early 1980s. Shinrin-yoku, also known as forest bathing, was a technique that was thought to reduce stress, albeit this wasn't proven. Since then, a wealth of data has demonstrated that spending time in nature is linked to several quantifiable health benefits in the body.

In an initial investigation, Yoshifumi Miyazaki, a specialist in forest therapy and researcher at Chiba University in Japan, discovered that individuals who strolled through a cedar forest for 40 minutes exhibited reduced levels of cortisol, a stress hormone linked to blood pressure and immune system performance, in contrast to those who walked in a lab setting. "I was taken aback," remembers Miyazaki. "Experiencing the forest fosters a feeling of physiological repose."

Similar to aromatherapy, which has also been studied for its therapeutic benefits, another researcher, Dr. Qing Li, a professor at the Nippon Medical School in Tokyo, discovered that aromatic compounds called phytoncides, which trees and plants emit, can, when inhaled, spur healthy biological changes. According to Li's research, persons who stroll through or spend the night in woods frequently have blood alterations linked to lowered blood pressure, improved immunity, and cancer prevention.

Studies conducted recently have also connected nature to the alleviation of symptoms related to heart disease, depression, cancer, anxiety, and attention deficit problems.

In the modern world, we frequently find ourselves cut off from nature due to the continual stimulation of technology and the bustle of metropolitan areas. On the other hand, empirical studies indicate that spending time in natural settings is extremely beneficial to our physical and mental health. The therapeutic benefits of nature are immense, whether one chooses to stroll through a park, climb through the mountains, or just relax by a peaceful lake.

What connection exists between wellbeing and nature? And how can you live a healthier life by bringing more nature into your life? Let's examine this in more depth below.

The connection between nature and physical health

Nature can encourage physical activity: being in nature encourages us to move our bodies, whether it's through a leisurely stroll or participating in outdoor activities like cycling, hiking, or swimming. A study found that engaging in physical exercise outside is significantly more likely to reduce the likelihood of experiencing poor mental health than engaging in physical activity indoors. Regular physical activity enhances strength, flexibility, and general physical well-being and assists in maintaining a healthy weight and cardiovascular fitness.

Nature enhances immune function: studies on the Japanese tradition of "forest bathing," or just spending time in the vicinity of trees, show that being in green areas improves the activity of natural killer cells and raises the synthesis of anti- inflammatory proteins, which strengthens the immune system. We get vitamin D from sunshine when we spend time outside, and vitamin D boosts and strengthens our immune system.

Nature reduces chronic disease risk: spending time in green areas has been linked by researchers to a lower risk of acquiring diseases, including diabetes, hypertension, and cardiovascular disease. Better general health results from physical exercise, lower stress levels, and cleaner air in natural settings.

The connection between nature and mental well-being

Because it offers a natural remedy for the stresses of daily life, nature helps people feel less stressed and anxious. Time spent in green areas is associated with lower cortisol levels, fewer anxiety symptoms, and more calm emotions. In summary, the calming influence of nature can assist in relieving the stress of contemporary life and restore mental equilibrium.

Happiness and mood are enhanced by nature: studies show that spending time in natural settings can improve happiness and mood while lowering depressive symptoms. All things considered, the combination of clean air, breathtaking scenery, and tranquility in nature is a powerful mood enhancer. Spending time in natural environments has been associated with increased creativity, focus, and problem-solving skills. Nature also improves cognitive function. Because nature offers a break from the never-ending stimulus of technology and urban settings, our minds may unwind and regenerate, which eventually improves cognitive function.

BOOK 3:

Nutrition for Healing

Nutrition for healing

L ong a supporter of a healthy diet, New York City Mayor Eric Adams recently launched six new plant-based lifestyle medicine initiatives across the city. In addition, he is urging everyone in New York to adopt a plant-based diet, which he began after being diagnosed with diabetes. After making the change, he claims that his energy level is "fantastic," his mental clarity has increased, and his health has improved. Consider being plant-based as a shift in lifestyle rather than a diet if that's what you want to do. "This way of thinking can contribute to gains in mental and physical health."

Plant-based diet

It is exactly what it sounds like—a plant-based diet. The main foods in the diet are plant-based foods, including fruits and vegetables, along with whole grains, legumes, nuts, and seeds.

A plant-based diet does not entail a vegetarian or vegan diet; instead, the majority of your nutrient intake should come from plant-based foods. You can still eat cattle, eggs, fish, chicken, and dairy products. A plant-based diet has no specific ratio of plant to animal products, although it's a good idea to start with eating at least two- thirds of each plate. Plants should receive the majority of attention.

These days, it's fashionable to use "plant-based diets" when discussing nutrition. Why? Charleston, South Carolina-based nutritionist Lauren Manaker, rd., believes it's because people are becoming more conscious of the advantages eating this way has for their health and the environment.

A portion of that might be attributed to documentaries like Cowspiracy (2014), game changers

(2018), and you are what you eat: a twin experiment (2024) that makes fun of consuming meat and other animal products.

However, what exactly does a "plant-based diet" entail? Is it synonymous with veganism or vegetarianism? Or does this diet merely need you to try to include more vegetables in your meals?

All of the aforementioned explanations are accurate in theory. "Some individuals mistakenly refer to a plant-based diet as a vegan diet." I've seen people use the word "plant-based" to refer to diets that consist largely, but not exclusively, of plant-based meals. Other people may use the term more broadly, encompassing all vegetarian diets.

How a plant-based diet works

Making plant-based foods the main component of your meals is the premise behind a plant-based diet. Easy enough, huh?

According to Manaker, "A plant-based diet limits things like meats, dairy, and eggs and emphasizes foods like fruits, vegetables, and beans." Afterward, more limitations could be imposed based on your desired level of strictness. "Depending on how each person interprets it, it may fully ban goods from animals or only limit intake," Manaker explains.

That means you could decide to reduce the amount of meat and fish you eat rather than making them off-limits entirely.

Different plant-based diet types

Consider the term "plant-based" as a general term that encompasses other, more specialized diets. For instance, Manaker claims that although the Mediterranean diet includes fish and poultry, its main focus is on plant-based meals, making it a form of a plant-based diet.

Among the plant-based diets are:

- Vegetarian

- Vegan

- Pesco vegetarian

- Semi-vegetarian or flexitarian

- Ovo vegetarian

- Lacto vegetarian

- Lacto-ovo vegetarian

- Raw vegan

Benefits of a plant-based diet

A review article found that the largest predictor of early death in the United States is having a poor-quality diet. When it comes to health and longevity, a traditional American diet heavy in processed meat, sodium, saturated and trans fats, and other unhealthy foods puts you at a disadvantage. On the other hand, a diet that emphasizes whole foods and plant-based nutrients seems to have the opposite effect. In fact, the majority of those who follow this eating pattern do so because they believe it may have health advantages. "Eating this way has been related to several cardiac advantages, including lower cholesterol," Manaker explains. "Eating a plant- based diet may improve reproductive indices and lower your risk of acquiring [type 2] diabetes, according to certain research." The academy of nutrition and dietetics states that everyone can safely follow a well- planned plant-based diet, including young children, newborns, and those who are pregnant or nursing.

As the data below indicates, eating a plant-based diet can help lower your chances of obesity and high blood pressure, help prevent or manage type 2 diabetes and heart disease, and possibly even lessen your need for medication. Here are some potential advantages of a plant-based diet in more detail.

Diminished chance of type 2 diabetes

A plant-based diet, which includes items like fruits, vegetables, legumes, nuts, and whole grains, was linked to a lower risk of type 2 diabetes, according to one review's findings. About 307,100 people participated in the nine trials, and the results were controlled for variables like exercise frequency and smoking status that might have had an impact on the findings. Thus, researchers concluded that the participants' dietary choices were responsible for the decreased risk.

The enhanced function of beta cells, which aid in the production of insulin (the hormone that maintains stable blood sugar levels), may be the cause of this decreased risk of type 2 diabetes. According to other studies, beta cell function decreases with the progression of type 2 diabetes, which can lead to potentially harmful variations in blood sugar levels.

However, after just 16 weeks on a plant-based diet, participants in a randomized trial showed improvements in their body mass index (BMI), reduced belly fat, and enhanced insulin sensitivity and beta cell activity when compared to the control group.

Manaker concurs that if you follow a plant-based diet in a healthy manner, it can help you manage your weight and possibly even help you lose weight. "Most individuals who switch from an American diet also notice an increase in energy," she continues.

Improved weight and blood sugar levels in diabetes patients

This diet is helpful for increasing metabolism, controlling weight, and decreasing inflammation, according to researchers from another study. It is especially good for persons who are obese and have type 1 and type 2 diabetes.

A plant-based diet has been linked to a lower risk of cancer and other chronic illnesses. The authors also noted evidence that indicated a plant-based diet may help prevent and manage type 2 diabetes. According to one review, patients with type 2 diabetes who follow a plant-based diet report better overall health, mental and physical well-being, and a higher quality of life. They also show improvements in physical markers of the disease.

A lower chance of heart problems

In one study, a diet high in plant-based foods (nuts, whole grains, fruits, vegetables, and oils) was found to reduce the risk of heart disease dramatically.

According to a different study, eating a diet high in plant-based foods and low in animal products was linked to a 16 percent lower risk of cardiovascular disease and a 31 to 32 percent lower risk of dying from it.

There are a number of things at work here, including the fact that a case study suggests that plant-based diets can reduce inflammation and cholesterol.

A lower cancer risk

Approximately 475,000 adults who were cancer-free at baseline were the subject of a UK study. A follow-up study conducted 11.4 years after the initial grouping of participants—vegetarians, low-meat eaters, fish eaters, and normal meat eaters— assessed their cancer incidence. Compared to habitual meat eaters, those who consumed less meat, ate fish, and were vegetarians had at lower risk of developing colorectal, breast, and prostate cancers. The lower cancer risk was thought to be partly attributed, according to the researchers, to having a low BMI.

In a separate study that was especially focused on breast cancer, it was discovered that those who adhered to a plant-based diet to the greatest extent were 67 percent less likely to get breast cancer than those who did not.

One thing to keep in mind: don't panic if you're not quite ready to give up animal proteins. According to other research, there is no higher risk linked to animal proteins, even though including more plant-based proteins in your diet can help reduce your risk of cardiovascular disease and cancer. Therefore, incorporating more plant-based proteins into your diet can still help reduce your risk of certain diseases, even if you don't have to fully give up dairy and meat. Manaker advises creating a grocery list that is primarily composed of vegetables, legumes, and plant-based proteins to ensure that you have plenty of options to choose from when you're hungry.

A plant-based diet may lower the risk of cancer and heart disease among black Americans, who are disproportionately impacted by several chronic diseases, according to one review.

An improved brain

A plant-based diet may benefit your physical and mental health. Although the evidence is conflicting, a study that included over 3,000 adults discovered that adhering to a plant-based diet was associated with improved cognitive function, particularly executive function and long-term memory. However, further research is needed to determine the exact mechanisms underlying these findings.

An extended life

According to several studies, a diet richer in plant protein is associated with a lower risk of premature death from all causes. According to one analysis, people who consumed the highest amounts of plant-based protein in their diets were 6% less likely to die young than those who ingested the least amount of protein overall. Increased consumption of fruits, vegetables, and legumes was linked to a decreased risk of dying young from all causes in one study involving 135,000 participants. The maximum health benefits were achieved at three to four servings per day, which is an amount that most people on a plant-based diet are likely to meet.

What to eat, limit, and avoid on a plant-based diet

What to eat and drink

- Vegetables

- Fruits

- Whole grains (such as quinoa, farro, brown rice, whole-wheat bread, and whole-wheat pasta)

- Beans

- Lentils

- Coffee

- Tea (including green, lavender, chamomile, or ginger)

What to limit (or avoid entirely)

- Dairy (including milk and cheese)

- Meat and poultry (like chicken, beef, and pork)

- All animal products (including eggs, dairy, and meat if you're following a vegan diet)

- Refined grains (such as "white" foods like white pasta, rice, and bread)

- Sweets (like cookies, brownies, and cake)

- Sweetened beverages, such as soda and fruit juice

- French fries

- Honey (if vegan)

How to transition

The following advice will help you get started:

Start out slowly

Making the switch to a vegan diet all at once is probably too drastic a shift to make in one sitting, but as with many significant endeavors, the key to success is to divide the task into manageable chunks.

Here are a few more suggestions to get you going. Perform these as fast or as slowly as you can bear, in any order:

Start by swapping out two foods that are derived from animals for healthier ones. Make a homemade cashew alfredo sauce instead of the conventional dairy version the next time you have pasta for dinner! Try a bean chili that is entirely plant-based instead of one that contains meat. Alternatively, replace the ground beef with sautéed tempeh (marinated in the same manner as your meat) on your next taco night.

Increase your intake of the fruits and vegetables you enjoy or have on hand. You can increase the amount of veggies on your plate each day or add fruit to smoothies and breakfast dishes.

Try introducing one or two different fruits and vegetables per week that you don't typically eat.

Every week, try a few different plant-based cuisines. Maybe a new bean or grain that you have never tried.

Replace processed meat-based meals like pizza, pasta, burgers, chicken nuggets, and sodas with plant-based substitutes. Try cooking a vegan cheese pizza at home with veggies, marinara, or cashew sauce instead of getting takeout. If you were a huge fan of these items, consider giving them up for one day each week in favor of a plant- based, less processed substitute.

Swap out your standard peanut butter for a natural one that has just nuts or seeds as the main ingredient and no additional sugar.

Try drinking infused water (water with pieces of real cucumber, strawberries, or blueberries) in place of soda.

If you haven't already, start preparing a couple of meals a week or cook more often at home instead of dining out. In addition to being expensive, fast food and restaurant meals frequently contain a lot of salt, oil, and added sugar to improve flavor and lengthen their shelf life. Your money and your health will both appreciate it if you cook more at home!

You will ultimately discover that you have abandoned many of your previous eating habits in favor of new, healthier ones as a result of making these small adjustments.

BOOK 4:

Exercise for Optimal Health

The power of exercise

You've likely heard the importance of exercise and are wondering why there's such a big deal. There are several scientifically supported reasons why becoming active can have a significant positive impact on your health; it's not just a fad. Exercise is a game-changer for many reasons, including how it can improve your mood and keep your body robust. Stay tuned if you're debating putting on those sneakers or simply want to know the ins and outs! We will discuss the many benefits of physical activity and why it ought to be an essential component of your daily regimen.

Exercise and health

Examining the history of exercise demonstrates how important it is to human survival and wellbeing. Physical activity used to be a natural part of people's daily routines, incorporated into work schedules and social norms rather than being a scheduled activity. From the martial arts of Africa to the yoga practices of India to the endurance running of the native Americans, this physical lifestyle was prevalent all across the world. Everyone agreed that exercise was essential for good health.

However, active lives started to decline as societies developed, especially with the transition to agricultural and later industrial ways of life. Over the past century, there has been a noticeable increase in the number of people leading sedentary lives. This change from an active to a sedentary lifestyle has had major negative effects on health. Our current state of inactivity is linked to a number of health problems, which supports the notion that regular physical activity is just as vital to our health as it was to our survival in the past.

Cardiovascular benefits: heart and blood vessels

Regular exercise is essential for maintaining heart health and controlling cardiovascular risk. Your heart works hard during exercise, which improves its ability to pump blood throughout your body. This effectiveness may help you control your stress and weight more effectively and lower your blood pressure. Additionally, exercise helps your body better utilize insulin, which protects your blood vessels against type 2 diabetes. Engaging in regular physical exercise can be likened to a cardiac tune-up, as it improves circulation, distributes oxygen and nutrients to critical areas, and reduces inflammation.

The type of exercise you choose can have an impact on your heart health in addition to other areas. Your heart and lungs get a boost from aerobic exercises like cycling or brisk walking, which directly supports heart-healthy exercise. On the other hand, strength exercises will increase bone and muscular strength and improve your body's general endurance. Don't forget the significance of flexibility and stretching either; these help preserve the health of your joints and enhance your general balance and coordination, all of which are beneficial for leading an active lifestyle. It has been demonstrated that even mild, contemplative motions from forms of exercise like tai chi can benefit those with hypertension and heart failure. Consequently, you lower your chance of heart disease and enhance your general health by including these various types of exercise.

Managing weight and metabolic process: maintaining balance on the scale

Exercise is essential for controlling weight and metabolism, which is particularly important for managing long-term illnesses like type 2 diabetes. Beyond the brief calorie burn during exercise, engaging in physical activity might trigger a metabolic surge. Because muscle tissue is an active metabolic player and uses more energy than fat tissue, regular exercise, especially strength training, can increase muscle mass and raise the resting metabolic rate. This will keep the energy expenditure scales tipped even when you're not working out. In addition to helping people control their weight, this is also helpful for those who have diabetes since it increases muscle cell's capacity to absorb glucose and use it as fuel, which helps control blood sugar levels. As a result, while exercise may not always result in weight loss, it is undeniably important for improving metabolism and maintaining a healthy weight.

For many chronic diseases associated with metabolic dysfunction, including but not limited to type 2 diabetes, regular exercise is an essential part of treatment. Because it has a positive impact on the metabolic function of various important tissues, physical activity is useful for weight control and metabolic health for a number of reasons.

For example, exercise lowers adipose tissue inflammation and fat mass, both of which are important components of insulin resistance, metabolic syndrome, and cardiovascular disorders. Additionally, it improves the liver's capacity to control blood sugar levels and the process by which food is converted into energy, thus promoting better metabolic health. The consequences are significant for those with chronic conditions: regular physical activity can enhance systemic inflammation and insulin sensitivity in the body, which are two major factors contributing to metabolic illnesses.

The gains in physiological function are observed in multiple metabolic regions, which may lower the likelihood of comorbidities linked to obesity and metabolic dysregulation. Thus, metabolic increases from exercise go hand in hand and offer a non-pharmacological way to manage and possibly even lessen the impact of long- term metabolic problems.

Mental health and cognitive clarity: the brain-exercise connection

Engaging in physical exercise provides significant protection against neurodegenerative illnesses and is a powerful tool for improving mood and mental clarity. Regular exercise improves mood and mental health in addition to bodily strength. Increases in neurotrophic factors, neurotransmitters, and hormones are the physiological response to exercise and are essential for the survival of neurons and the promotion of neuroplasticity. Physical activity turns the brain into a growing, healing environment that supports processes like angiogenesis, neurogenesis, and synaptic plasticity—all of which reinforce neural networks.

Furthermore, regular physical activity has a profound positive impact on neurological health, especially for people who are at risk of developing Parkinson's or Alzheimer's disease. Studies have shown that those who incorporate physical activity into their daily routine have a reduction in the risk factors linked to these illnesses. A symbiotic relationship between the autonomic and central nervous systems is fostered by the reverberating effects of exercise on the nervous system at large. Maintaining this equilibrium is essential for maintaining cognitive abilities, which are frequently weakened in neurodegenerative illnesses. In addition to preventing the outward signs of aging, exercise protects the complex circuitry of the brain by acting as a barrier against the development and worsening of cognitive deficits.

Exercise to prolong your life: delaying the aging process

Scientific studies are progressively revealing the connection between aging and exercise. Regular physical activity has been linked to a longer lifespan and fewer signs of aging, according to thorough assessments of numerous studies. Frequent exercise has been associated with a significantly lower risk of numerous serious illnesses, including heart disease, stroke, type 2 diabetes, hypertension, and several cancers. Furthermore, when comparing physically active people to their inactive counterparts, a regular exercise regimen has been linked to an approximate 30% to 35% decrease in all-cause mortality.

Research has made an effort to measure how much exercise affects life expectancy. According to research, those who engage in regular physical activity may live an extra 0.4 to almost 7 years, depending on their circumstances. This increase is sustained even when other mortality risk factors are taken into consideration. There is diversity when it comes to various forms of physical exercise, especially when considering that these assessments do not account for mortality risk variables despite the research regularly demonstrating longer life expectancies in athletes with aerobic endurance. When examining the various forms of exercise, a combination of moderate and intense physical activity seems to be the most advantageous. 150–300 minutes of moderate exercise or 75–150 minutes of strenuous exercise per week are suggested per the recommended guidelines. Exceeding these suggestions, nevertheless, might have even more advantages. For example, those who exercised moderately for 300 to 599 minutes a week reduced their all-cause mortality by 26% to 31%, but those who exercised more vigorously than recommended experienced a reduction of 21% to 23%.

The fact that long-term moderate and intense physical activity has advantages for people of all ages must also be emphasized. Although younger people might choose more strenuous sports, elderly people still enjoy moderate exercise because it benefits longevity. This implies that exercise can be customized to an individual's skills and yet have a major positive impact on health, in addition to helping to slow down the aging process.

Exercise Regimens that promote healing

If you've never exercised before, you might want to experiment with various forms of exercise to see what suits you best. Recall that you should consider the type of movement you enjoy doing in addition to your range of motion. You're more inclined to stick with something you enjoy doing. Additionally, you may enjoy different kinds of exercise. Adding diverse types of physical activities to your exercise regimen actually helps you target different muscle groups in different ways.

Cardio

Cardiovascular exercise, sometimes known as aerobic exercise, is any type of physical activity that raises your heart rate, pumps blood, and activates your lungs. In addition to enhancing the health of your entire body and mind, it stimulates and fortifies your cardiovascular system. Cardio can reduce stress, enhance sleep quality, and release endorphins into your brain. It's also a really useful tool for losing weight. Cardio is one of the easiest and most accessible types of exercise. As long as you start to feel hot, sweaty, and out of breath, a vigorous stroll or yard labor can be considered aerobic exercise. Although the stereotypical picture of cardio is someone puffing while running, there are a plethora of options available for cardio exercises: Strolling and trekking: since it can be done practically anyplace and requires minimal equipment, walking is one of the best aerobic exercises available. All you need is a good pair of supportive yet comfy sneakers. Start by walking for five to ten minutes daily, then gradually increase that time to thirty minutes or longer. Walking on a regular basis can strengthen your bones and muscles, lower your risk of disease, lift your spirits, and help you lose weight. Hiking involves steeper, more uneven trails than walking, but it also often burns more calories because it lets you explore and enjoy nature. Furthermore, studies indicate that simply being outside has several health advantages.

Running

All you need to start running, just like walking, is a pair of shoes that fit properly. Regular running can enhance your emotional, physical, and cardiovascular well-being regardless of speed or location. Stepping out: try dancing for an engaging and enjoyable workout. Dancing can improve your cardiovascular health in the same ways as other forms of exercise, but it can also help you become more flexible as you learn new body movements. Not to mention that mastering the choreography and the social components of dancing improves our cognitive abilities.

Cycling

Cycling is a fantastic method to work your heart and lungs while strengthening and toning your lower body. Additionally, riding a stationary bike and maintaining your upright position improves your posture and balance. Another excellent substitute for driving, one of our most common sedentary activities, is riding a bike. Try riding your bike the next time you have somewhere to go—like the grocery store, a friend's house, or the post office.

Swimming

All the cardiovascular advantages of aerobic exercise without any of the impact are obtained by swimming. Engaging in aquatic exercise provides a respite for your joints while simultaneously fortifying all of your body's muscles. Also, you can burn calories without perspiring as much.

Nothing raises your heart rate more than jumping rope. You can fit this highly effective cardiovascular exercise into any hectic schedule. Ten to fifteen minutes of jumping rope is all you need to obtain the heart-healthy benefits you require. It's also enjoyable!

Strength training

Gaining muscle and reducing fat can be achieved through strength training. This kind of exercise entails applying resistance to your muscles by pushing against gravity or lifting and moving large things. Strength training comes in a plethora of ways, contingent on your equipment and level of weightlifting.

Exercises using body weight exercises that only require your body weight are typically sufficient to become stronger when you first start strength training. Burpees, lunges, squats, planks, and pushups are all excellent choices. You can also practice and perfect appropriate technique by performing these workouts without adding weight, which is crucial for avoiding future injuries.

Scales: before lifting weights on your own, you might have extra opportunities to hone your form using weight machines. Additionally, you can use machines to target particular muscles and get a more controlled range of motion.

Free weights: performing functional exercises, such as lifting weights, can improve your ability to perform everyday tasks like carrying groceries, climbing stairs, and housecleaning. The complete muscle group training improves strength, balance, and coordination.

All three of these categories of weight-related exercise can be combined into a full strength training program.

Stretching

Stretching improves and preserves your body's flexibility or capacity to move in many directions without risk of harm. Regular stretching can improve your physical performance, allow you to use your entire range of motion, and help you prevent accidents. Although stretching is most beneficial right after a workout when your muscles are warmed up from movement, it may be done at any time.

Stretching that is static involves stretching your muscles as far as they will go without causing you any pain and then keeping that position for a period of 15 to 30 seconds. Static stretching comes in two flavors: active and passive. When you stretch actively, you tighten one muscle to release tension in the other. Your hamstrings can stretch and lengthen while your thigh muscles tense when you raise your leg straight up into the air while lying on your back. During passive stretching, you assist your body in extending by using an external push, such as your hand. A passive stretch for your thigh muscle is when you bend your knee and hold your foot behind you with your hand.

Dynamic stretching: to get your muscles warmed up and prepared for action, consider dynamic stretching before a workout. Stretching dynamically involves more movement than simply touching your toes. Toe touches, high knees, butt kicks, and lateral shuffles are among the motions.

Consult a physical therapist or your doctor if stretching causes you pain. They can recommend painless stretches that will gradually improve your range of motion.

Exercises for balance

As you age, maintaining your balance becomes even more crucial for a variety of sports and everyday activities. Improving your balance today will help you avoid falls later in life and the injuries they frequently cause.

Yoga: numerous benefits of yoga include improved flexibility, improved sleep, and improved happiness. Balance is a major component of any yoga practice. Yoga puts your body through a variety of dynamic poses and situations that test its ability to maintain balance. By doing this, you strengthen those vital stabilizing muscles and loosen up tense muscles, both of which reduce your chance of falling.

Tai chi: tai chi is a low-impact exercise that is very portable and very effective at reducing stress and enhancing balance. You can practice shifting your weight from one foot to another with your arms outstretched thanks to the flowing movements from one pose to the next.

BOOK 5:

Essentials of Natural Healing

One of the most significant lessons we've learned in the medical field is: As usual, the most crucial thing we can do to enhance our health is to concentrate on the fundamentals.

We cannot get good health; it is something we must cultivate and preserve. Consider it like this: before starting to build a house, builders take great care to ensure that the foundation is sturdy and firm. In the same way, we cannot expect to improve our health if we do not first lay some fundamental groundwork.

Importance of water and hydration

The basis of life is hydration. We just cannot exist without it. We must maintain our body's water content, which ranges from 60 to 80 percent, by drinking enough water. Rehydrating our bodies involves restoring the water lost through perspiration, urine, and other physiological processes. We will discuss the advantages of maintaining hydration as well as the reasons it is so crucial in this section.

Regulates body temperature

Temperature regulation is one of the main roles that water plays in the body. Sweating helps us cool off when we get too heated. As the water in our perspiration evaporates, an electrolyte imbalance results, which removes heat from our skin and aids in controlling our body temperature. We won't sweat enough to maintain a healthy body temperature if we don't drink enough electrolyte-rich water, which increases the risk of heat exhaustion and possibly heatstroke.

Aids in digestion

Digestion also benefits from enough hydration. Water aids in the digestion and passage of food via our digestive systems. We risk experiencing constipation and stomach pain if we don't drink enough water. Maintaining a healthy digestive tract and preventing constipation may be achieved by consuming enough water.

Improves cognitive function

According to research, maintaining proper hydration helps enhance cognitive abilities such as concentration, thinking, and attention. This is because electrolytes are necessary for the brain to operate correctly. Our brains don't work at their peak when we are dehydrated, which can cause headaches, exhaustion, and trouble focusing. Increasing our intake of electrolyte-rich water can aid in enhancing cognitive performance and increase productivity.

Helps to flush toxins

When it comes to eliminating poisons from our systems, water is essential. Water is necessary for our kidneys to filter waste and poisons out of our blood, which is subsequently expelled as urine. Toxins may accumulate in our bodies as a result of our kidneys' inability to work correctly if we don't drink enough water. By staying hydrated, we can keep these poisons out of our systems and maintain healthy kidney function.

Improves athletic performance

It's critical for athletes and everyone participating in physical exercise to stay hydrated. Sweating during exercise causes our body to lose water. Insufficient consumption of water or electrolyte-free water can result in dehydration, which can cause exhaustion, cramping in the muscles, and even heatstroke. Taking a hydration enhancer before, during, and after exercise can assist in avoiding dehydration and enhance athletic performance.

Helps to maintain healthy skin

For skin to be healthy, one must be hydrated. Nudge keeps our skin firm and moisturized, which helps minimize the look of wrinkles and fine lines. Additionally, it aids in the removal of toxins from the skin, helping to ward off acne and other skin issues. Our skin might become dry and lifeless if we don't drink enough water, which can make us appear older than we actually are.

Prevents headaches

Headaches are frequently caused by dehydration. Headaches and migraines can result from our brains not functioning correctly when we are thirsty. Our brains work best when we are well-hydrated, and drinking lots of water can help avoid headaches.

In summary, maintaining proper hydration is critical to our health and wellbeing. It aids in temperature regulation, digestion, enhances mental clarity, eliminates toxins, enhances physical performance, keeps skin healthy, and avoids headaches. To stay well hydrated during the day, drinking a lot of water is important. Try adding a nudge hydration enhancer to your water if it lacks essential electrolytes for flavor and to encourage you to drink plenty of water. Recall that a healthy body is one that is well hydrated!

How the body detoxes

Now that we are aware of the kinds of toxins that our bodies are frequently exposed to, let's examine how the body eliminates them. This section delineates the function of each organ in the detoxification process without delving too far into the science.

The liver

Consider the liver to be your primary detoxifier. It functions as a filter, taking out toxins that are produced by our body during regular metabolism. These harmful byproducts are broken down by the liver and subsequently eliminated by the kidneys. Additionally, it aids in the body's removal of external pollutants like alcohol, narcotics, chemicals, and heavy metals as well as infections like bacteria and viruses, cholesterol, and hormones.

The kidneys

The kidneys serve as a filter, much like the liver does. They remove waste and unwanted materials from our bodies, including hazardous chemicals and pharmaceutical byproducts. The kidneys also maintain the proper balance of fluids and electrolytes in our bodies. This is essential for keeping the ph balance of your body, enabling cell activity, and regulating blood pressure.

The digestive tract

Supporting detoxification is one of the digestive tract's many functions. Through bowel movements, the digestive tract aids in the removal of poisons. This necessitates sustaining optimal intestinal health by consuming adequate fiber and tending to the billions of microbes residing within our stomachs. The consumption of fiber derived from whole-food plant-based sources functions as a filler in the digestive system, aiding in the removal of toxins, heavy metals, and excess hormones. Along with assisting in the reduction of dangerous bacterial and yeast overgrowth, it also maintains the beneficial bacteria in the gut.

The lymphatic system

The fluid that permeates the whole body is called lymph. It is a component of the immune system as a whole, whose main job is to keep foreign substances out of our bodies and shield our cells from them. The tonsils, spleen, thymus, and adenoids are all parts of the lymphatic system, which comprises hundreds of lymph nodes and a network of capillaries and veins. This special system is crucial to detoxification because it carries white blood cells, also known as lymphocytes, which aid in the body's defense against toxins and diseases.

The respiratory system

The tiny hairs within your nostrils, starting with the nose, act as a barrier to help keep dust and other pollutants out of your lungs. Your nose and lungs produce mucus, which forms a second layer of defense. Lastly, the lungs and bronchi assist in the conversion of poisons into carbonic gas (CO_2), which is exhaled when you breathe in oxygen.

The skin

Consider the skin to be the body's first line of protection. The skin, which is the biggest organ in the body, acts as a barrier to keep out harmful chemicals, germs, and viruses. Sweating is another way that the skin permits the detoxification process to take place.

Even while the liver and kidneys carry out the majority of the heavy work during detoxification, they can't always eliminate all the toxins. What remains is kept in reserve as fat. Through this secondary system, the body is able to eliminate pollutants such as heavy metals, arsenic, lead, and mercury through sweating.

Water detox

Consider detoxifying your body as a kind of spring cleaning. Eliminate the undesirable and accentuate the positive.

In recent years, detoxification has become increasingly popular. However, what does it actually imply, and how can consuming water support your attempts to improve your health? Before we answer those queries, let's take a quick look at history.

Detoxing has roots in native American, Greek, and Roman traditions that span several millennia. Despite the differences in their approaches, they all aimed to rid their bodies of poisons and undesirable substances. The aim has been and continues to be overall health.

Nowadays, it's impossible to enter a pharmacy or grocery shop without seeing hundreds of detox solutions that promise to remove undesirable substances from your body. However, water detox is one of the greatest (and healthiest) detoxes you can do at home.

The water detox

Water is a vital component of life, and it is also necessary for optimum health. One of the simplest methods to keep your body healthy and prevent weariness and dehydration is drinking water daily. Numerous other advantageous health effects are also present.

Creating a strategy is the first step in attempting a water detox. If you perform a water detox properly, the advantages become apparent quickly, even if it won't be simple. The idea is to temporarily boost your fluid intake in order to alleviate bloating and remove toxins from your system. Here are some guidelines:

Keep it brief: it's better to give it a few days. It is not something you want to do to your body what it needs. If you overdo it, the advantages of the detox may be lost since you will likely overeat when it is finished.

Have a lot of filtered, cold water to drink. Try these suggestions for boosting your water consumption if you are finding it difficult to meet your objectives.

Add some fruits and vegetables with a high water content to your h20. In addition to the health benefits of water, the meal contains vitamins and antioxidants. Green leafy veggies and watermelon are excellent places to start.

Make a note of the things you see becoming better to help you stay motivated. Your skin, energy, weight decrease, etc. This will clarify the advantages of detox for you and demonstrate why it was beneficial.

Sunshine: nature's healer

Contemporary beliefs typically paint the sun in a negative way. It's common knowledge that we should shield ourselves from the sun and use sunscreen whenever we go outside. Although sunburn and melanoma are two major health issues associated with sun exposure, the fact remains that sun exposure in moderation can be therapeutic due to the sun's remarkable health advantages. Furthermore, current studies indicate that individuals with certain disorders, such as cancer, have a lower chance of surviving if they receive insufficient sun exposure. Sun exposure treatment is becoming increasingly popular as more individuals come to understand the therapeutic benefits of sunlight.

History of sunlight therapy

The sun has been revered for its amazing healing properties in many different cultures throughout history. Therefore, humanity has been aware of the sun's health benefits since prehistoric times. The Vedas, an old and revered Hindu text, acknowledges sun treatment as a potent natural remedy for several health issues. The sun is an essential element of Indian culture. In reality, people in India still use sacred sun salutations like Surya Namaskar, which are believed to have healing properties for the physical, psychological, and spiritual domains.

According to the ancient Roman scholar Pliny, the sun is the most significant natural self-administered remedy. Hippocrates and other well-known medical professionals from Arabia and Rome lauded the inherent therapeutic benefits of heliotherapy, which is the use of sunlight for certain skin disorders. Epilepsy, asthma, obesity, jaundice, and disorders of the colon and bladder were all treated with sunlight treatment under the Roman Empire. Rickets and scurvy were known to be alleviated by sunlight in the 1700s. In the late 1800s, cholera, anthrax, and dysentery were among the bacterial illnesses for which the sun was known to be beneficial. Renowned sunlight therapists Koch and Finsen were awarded the Nobel Prize in 1903 and 1905, respectively, for their innovative use of UV light in the treatment of tuberculosis.

For more than 40 years, Dr. Auguste Rollier of Switzerland effectively treated tuberculosis with sun therapy. Of the 2,167 patients, 1,746 received successful treatment; the other patients' failures were limited to further advanced cases. Florence Nightingale was employed by a number of institutions in the early 1900s to improve the healing effects of sunlight. Dr. Oskar Bernhard used sun therapy to treat wounds and prevent tetanus and gangrene during World War I. The sun's possible health benefits were eventually acknowledged.

The neural, skin, circulatory, musculoskeletal, respiratory, and circulatory systems were all treated with sunlight therapy throughout the 1900s. However, natural therapeutic methods like sunlight treatment have gradually been supplanted since the development of medicines like penicillin.

Vitamin d synthesis

The first rays of morning sunlight gently rouse you from sleep by stimulating the creation of serotonin and cortisol. More serotonin is released throughout the day as the retina senses sunlight.

Serotonin controls appetite and elevates mood. When night falls, serotonin is converted to melatonin, which promotes sleep. To ensure that you wake up feeling rejuvenated, you should minimize the use of electronic displays at night and leave your curtains open to let in early sunlight. The generation of vitamin D also depends on sunlight.

A healthy level of vitamin D is linked to happier moods on its own, but research has also shown that sun exposure in large amounts can lower levels of depression and weariness regardless of vitamin D status. In winter, you're not the only one who feels depressed. Depression, known as seasonal affective disorder, typically develops in response to a shift in the seasons, primarily the decrease in sunlight that occurs throughout the winter. Enkephalin, beta-endorphin, and adrenocorticotropic hormone can all be produced when exposed to sunlight. These compounds protect the heart, inhibit pain, and lower stress. Because beta-endorphin has an opiate-like impact on the brain, it may be addictive and cause withdrawal symptoms when sun exposure is reduced.

Spend at least 30 minutes a day in the sun, with at least your arms and legs exposed, to make sure you're getting enough vitamin D.

In a long-term study including Swedish women, it was discovered that while deliberately avoiding the sun lowered life expectancy and raised the risk of cardiovascular disease, sun-seeking behavior was linked to an increased risk of skin malignancies but did not affect life expectancy. Even smokers who had a lot of sun exposure outlived non-smokers who stayed out of the sun.

Both vitamin D and sunshine are good for heart health. The sun's ultraviolet (UVA) rays cause the synthesis of nitric oxide, which controls fluid balance and blood pressure. Winter is associated with a higher risk of coronary heart disease, stroke, and possibly fatal blood clots than summer. In actuality, winter death rates are far higher than summer ones in the majority of affluent nations, including Australia.

At the equator, where there is an abundance of sunshine, the incidence of type 1 diabetes in children is lowest and correlates with latitude. While excessive amounts of melatonin, which are created when there is no sunlight, can hinder the manufacturing of insulin, vitamin D reduces the chance of developing type 2 diabetes. A sign of improper blood sugar control, glycated hemoglobin levels are often significantly lower in the summer than in the winter.

When exposed to sunlight, alpha-melanocyte-stimulating hormone is created, which controls glucose metabolism, reduces appetite, and increases libido. Independent of vitamin D levels, sunlight has also been shown to enhance the quality of your gut flora and lower the risk of inflammatory bowel disease. Research suggests that exposure to sunlight can have numerous health benefits, including enhancing mitochondrial function, mitigating acne, preventing cancer, and promoting bone health and autoimmune disorders via generating vitamin D.

The sunshine vitamin

Fat-soluble vitamin D stimulates the body's defenses against illness. It is necessary for the parathyroid glands to regulate blood calcium levels and for intestinal calcium absorption. About 25% of Australians do not get enough vitamin D, and the percentage rises during the colder months. A lack of vitamin D can lead to a variety of health problems, including delayed physical development in children and babies, gut dysfunction, softening of the teeth and bones, cardiac problems, and seasonal affective disorder. Nervousness, diarrhea, burning in the mouth and throat, nearsightedness, muscle weakness, and cramps are among the deficiency's warning signs and symptoms. Iron deficiency, raised serum phosphatase, elevated follicle- stimulating hormone, and elevated parathyroid hormone levels are frequently associated with vitamin D inadequacy. Childhood rickets, a softening of the bones characterized by severe instances characterized by bowed legs, is caused by an absolute deficiency.

The steroid 7-dehydrocholesterol is secreted onto the surface of your skin by oil glands in order to produce vitamin D. Precholecalciferol is created when this is reabsorbed into the skin's outer layers and combines with ultraviolet b (UVB) radiation. After that, the precholecalciferol must be reorganized over the course of two to three days in order to generate vitamin d3, also known as cholecalciferol. This molecule enters your bloodstream through the skin and diffuses, traveling to various parts of your body where it acts.

Spend at least 30 minutes a day in the sun, with at least your arms and legs exposed, to make sure you're getting enough vitamin D. To prevent sunburn, this should happen before 10 a.m. Or after 2 p.m. In the Australian summer. The same dose will take longer to receive on cloudy or low-uv days. It is nearly impossible to pinpoint the precise amount of sunshine you require because it depends on your latitude, altitude, complexion, and daily weather fluctuations.

Health benefits of the sun

The following is a summary of some of the incredible abilities of sunlight: Prevents insufficiency of vitamin D

Vitamin D is essential for healthy teeth and bones, boosts immunity, and aids in the battle against depression. Vitamin D insufficiency has been associated with less exposure to sunlight.

You may be more susceptible to osteoporosis, autoimmune illnesses, depression, cancer, chronic pain, and weak muscles if you have low vitamin D levels. Since vitamin D is found in very few foods, exposure to sunlight is the most effective way to absorb this essential vitamin. Your body will produce more vitamin D with moderate sunlight exposure.

Combats stress and sleeplessness

Anxiety, despair, insomnia, and an inability to eat well are all possible signs of afs. The hormone serotonin is essential for controlling mood, appetite, and sleep patterns. Recovering from adrenal fatigue requires getting adequate restorative sleep. It's time to give your body some sunshine and put an end to those antidepressants loaded with chemicals. Elevated levels of sunlight exposure stimulate the creation of serotonin, which in turn improves mood, reduces stress, increases appetite, and improves sleep.

Provides relief from skin disorders

It's well known that sunlight has extraordinary healing properties. Natural sunlight's ultraviolet radiation can help with skin disorders such as psoriasis, acne, scleroderma, atopic dermatitis, eczema, and jaundice.

Aids rheumatoid arthritis and osteoporosis

In addition to being recognized to induce rheumatoid arthritis, vitamin D insufficiency is a major contributing factor to osteoporosis, an age-related condition characterized by weak, brittle bones. Rheumatoid arthritis can be debilitating in severe cases. Research has indicated a higher incidence of rheumatoid arthritis in higher latitudes—where sunlight is scarcer—than in lower latitudes, which are closer to the equator. Furthermore, the longer a person is exposed to sunlight, the worse off they are from the sickness.

Exposure to sunlight stimulates your body's production of vitamin D and facilitates the absorption of calcium and phosphorus, which are vital for strong bones and teeth. As a result, sunlight can offer some relief from ailments like osteoporosis and rheumatoid arthritis while also preventing high blood pressure, stroke, and heart attacks.

Helps fight seasonal affective disorder

Depression, known as seasonal affective disorder (sad), typically starts in early fall and gets worse in the winter. Deficits in vitamin D and sunlight are recognized to be the disorder's causes. Sunshine exposure can help alleviate seasonal affective disorder (sad) by increasing vitamin D and serotonin, also referred to as the "happy hormone."

Maintains your circadian rhythm

Your body's circadian cycle depends on the sun, which is one of the sun's many health benefits. Your body and mind need hormones to work correctly, which sunlight helps to regulate. This synchronizes your circadian rhythm. Moreover, UV light exposure causes the body to produce melatonin, a potent antioxidant that aids in the fight against cancer.

Additional health benefits of the sun

Sun exposure helps heal wounds, lower mortality rates, alleviate infant jaundice, control body temperature, lessen chronic discomfort and body odor, and aid in the battle against persistent weight gain. The retina, which is found at the back of the eye, receives natural sunlight, which aids in synchronizing your body's vital biorhythms.

BOOK 6:

Herbal Treatments with Ailment

Solutions

Renowned for her proficiency in natural health and holistic wellness, Dr. Barbara O'Neill is a naturopath, author, and health educator. Dr. O'Neill has devoted her professional life to teaching people how to use natural remedies and lifestyle modifications to enhance their body's innate healing capabilities. She has decades of experience in the field.

Her journey started with a strong interest in nutrition and health, which inspired her to pursue in-depth research, naturopathy training, and wellness education. Dr. O'Neill rose to prominence in the natural health community as a result of her dedication to comprehending the complex relationships between diet, lifestyle, and health.

Dr. O'Neill has reached a global audience through her books, many seminars, workshops, and online courses throughout her career. She places a strong emphasis on stress reduction, regular exercise, detoxification, and a plant-based diet in her teachings. She is a fervent supporter of utilizing natural treatments in place of processed foods and dangerous chemicals.

Among Dr. O'neill's accomplishments are her numerous recommendations for practical and understandable health improvement. Many people have been motivated by her work to take control of their health by making wise, healthy decisions. She continues to change people's lives by sharing her knowledge and enthusiasm for holistic health as a committed educator, helping them lead healthier, more balanced live

The comprehensive guide to over 800 ailments and their natural remedies

1. Abdominal aortic aneurysm = take hawthorn, consume hawthorn berry tea or supplements to support cardiovascular health. Dosage: drink 1 cup of hawthorn berry tea 2-3 times daily or take 250-500 mg of hawthorn supplements twice daily.

2. Abdominal pain = take ginger, chew raw ginger or make a tea from fresh ginger slices to help manage abdominal pain. Dosage: chew 1-2 slices of raw ginger or drink 1 cup of ginger tea 2-3 times daily.

3. Abortion (post-procedure recovery) = use raspberry leaf, and drink raspberry leaf tea to support uterine health and recovery. Dosage: drink 1 cup of raspberry leaf tea 2-3 times daily.

4. Acanthosis nigricans = take turmeric, apply turmeric paste topically, and consume turmeric supplements to reduce skin darkening. Dosage: apply turmeric paste once daily and take 400-600 mg of turmeric supplements 3 times daily.

5. Achalasia = use peppermint, use peppermint and drink peppermint tea to help relax the esophagus and ease swallowing. Dosage: drink 1 cup of peppermint tea 2-3 times daily.

6. Achalasia & swallowing disorder = take peppermint, make a tea from dried peppermint leaves to help relax the esophagus. Dosage: drink 1 cup of peppermint tea 2-3 times daily.

7. Acid and chemical burns = apply aloe vera, apply aloe vera gel topically to soothe and heal burns. Dosage: apply aloe vera gel 2-3 times daily.

8. Acid reflux & heartburn = take ginger, chew raw ginger or make a tea from fresh ginger slices to help manage acid reflux and heartburn. Dosage: chew 1-2 slices of raw ginger or drink 1 cup of ginger tea 2-3 times daily.

9. Acid reflux in babies = use chamomile,, give chamomile tea in small amounts to soothe the digestive tract. Dosage: give 1-2 teaspoons of chamomile tea 1-2 times daily.

10. Acne = take tea tree oil, apply diluted tea tree oil to affected areas for acne treatment. Dosage: apply 5% diluted tea tree oil once daily.

11. Acoustic neuroma (vestibular schwannoma) = use ginkgo biloba, take ginkgo biloba supplements to improve circulation and support nerve health. Dosage: take 120-240 mg of ginkgo biloba supplements 1-2 times daily.

12. Acromegaly = take reishi mushroom, consume reishi mushroom supplements to help balance hormone levels. Dosage: take 1,000-1,500 mg of reishi mushroom supplements 2-3 times daily.

13. Actinic keratoses (solar keratoses) = apply green tea extract, apply green tea extract topically to reduce skin lesions. Dosage: apply green tea extract 2-3 times daily.

14. Actinomycosis = use garlic, consume raw garlic or garlic supplements to fight bacterial infections. Dosage: consume 2-3 raw garlic cloves daily or take 600-1,200 mg of garlic supplements daily.

15. Acupuncture (post-treatment support) = take ginger, drink ginger tea to reduce inflammation and support recovery. Dosage: drink 1 cup of ginger tea 2-3 times daily.

16. Acute bronchitis & chest congestion = take thyme, make a tea from dried thyme leaves to help manage bronchitis. Dosage: drink 1 cup of thyme tea 2-3 times daily.

17. Acute cholecystitis = use dandelion root, drink dandelion root tea to support liver and gallbladder health. Dosage: drink 1 cup of dandelion root tea 2-3 times daily.

18. Acute kidney injury = take nettle, consume nettle tea to support kidney function and reduce inflammation. Dosage: drink 1 cup of nettle tea 2-3 times daily.

19. Acute lymphoblastic leukemia = use astragalus, take astragalus supplements to support the immune system. Dosage: take 250-500 mg of astragalus supplements 2-3 times daily.

20. Acute myeloid leukaemia = take milk thistle, consume milk thistle supplements to support liver function during treatment. Dosage: take 150-300 mg of milk thistle supplements 2-3 times daily.

21. Acute pancreatitis = use turmeric, take turmeric supplements to reduce inflammation and support pancreatic health. Dosage: take 400-600 mg of turmeric supplements 3 times daily.

22. Acute respiratory distress syndrome (ards) = take elecampane, drink elecampane tea to support respiratory health. Dosage: drink 1 cup of elecampane tea 2-3 times daily.

23. Addison's disease = use licorice root, consume licorice root tea to support adrenal gland function. Dosage: drink 1 cup of licorice root tea 1-2 times daily.

24. Addison's disease & adrenal insufficiency = take licorice root, consume licorice root tea or supplements to support adrenal function and manage addison's disease. Dosage: drink 1 cup of licorice root tea 1-2 times daily or take 300-600 mg of licorice root supplements daily.

25. Adenoidectomy (post-surgery recovery) = take calendula, apply calendula cream to reduce inflammation and support healing. Dosage: apply calendula cream 2-3 times daily.

26. Adenomyosis = use ginger, drink ginger tea to reduce menstrual pain and inflammation. Dosage: drink 1 cup of ginger tea 2-3 times daily.

27. Age spots & hyperpigmentation = take lemon juice, apply fresh lemon juice to age spots to help lighten them. Dosage: apply lemon juice to affected areas once daily.

28. Agoraphobia & anxiety = take passionflower, make a tea from dried passionflower leaves or consume passionflower supplements to help manage anxiety. Dosage: drink 1 cup of passionflower tea 2-3 times daily or take 200-400 mg of passionflower supplements daily.

29. Agranulocytosis & low white blood cells = take astragalus, consume astragalus supplements to help support white blood cell production. Dosage: take 500-1,000 mg of astragalus supplements 2-3 times daily.

30. Aids = take echinacea, consume echinacea supplements or make a tea from dried echinacea roots to support immune function in aids. Dosage: take 300-500 mg of echinacea supplements 2-3 times daily or drink 1 cup of echinacea tea 2-3 times daily.

31. Alcohol poisoning = use milk thistle, take milk thistle supplements to support liver detoxification and recovery. Dosage: take 150-300 mg of milk thistle supplements 2-3 times daily.

32. Alcohol withdrawal syndrome & delirium tremens = take kudzu, consume kudzu root extract or supplements to help manage symptoms of alcohol withdrawal and delirium tremens. Dosage: take 1,000-1,500 mg of kudzu root supplements daily.

33. Alcohol-related liver disease = take dandelion root, consume dandelion root tea to support liver health and function. Dosage: drink 1 cup of dandelion root tea 2-3 times daily.

34. Alcoholism = take kudzu root, consume kudzu root supplements to help manage alcohol cravings and support recovery from alcoholism. Dosage: take 1,000-1,500 mg of kudzu root supplements daily.

35. Alexander technique (post-session support) = use chamomile, drink chamomile tea to relax muscles and reduce tension. Dosage: drink 1 cup of chamomile tea 2-3 times daily.

36. Alkaptonuria = take turmeric, consume turmeric supplements to reduce inflammation and support joint health. Dosage: take 400-600 mg of turmeric supplements 3 times daily.

37. Allergic rhinitis = use stinging nettle, drink stinging nettle tea to alleviate allergy symptoms. Dosage: drink 1 cup of stinging nettle tea 2-3 times daily.

38. Allergic rhinitis & hay fever = take nettle, make a tea from dried nettle leaves or consume nettle supplements to help alleviate allergic rhinitis and hay fever symptoms. Dosage: drink 1 cup of nettle tea 2-3 times daily or take 300-600 mg of nettle supplements daily.

39. Allergies = take nettle, steep dried leaves in hot water for 10-15 minutes to make a tea for allergy relief. Dosage: drink 1 cup of nettle tea 2-3 times daily.

40. Alopecia areata & hair loss = take rosemary, apply rosemary oil to the scalp or make a tea from dried rosemary leaves to help stimulate hair growth and manage alopecia areata. Dosage: apply rosemary oil to the scalp 2-3 times weekly or drink 1 cup of rosemary tea daily.

41. Alport syndrome = use nettle to support kidney health. Dosage: drink 1 cup of nettle tea 2-3 times daily or take 300-600 mg of nettle supplements daily.

42. Altitude sickness & hypoxia = take ginkgo biloba, make a tea from dried ginkgo biloba leaves or consume ginkgo biloba supplements to help manage altitude sickness and hypoxia. Dosage: drink 1 cup of ginkgo biloba tea 2-3 times daily or take 120-240 mg of ginkgo biloba supplements daily.

43. Alzheimer's disease = take turmeric, use turmeric powder in cooking or make a tea with turmeric and black pepper for anti-inflammatory effects to potentially benefit cognitive function in alzheimer's disease. Dosage: take 400-600 mg of turmeric supplements 3 times daily or add 1 teaspoon of turmeric powder with a pinch of black pepper to meals daily.

44. Amblyopia = take bilberry, consume bilberry supplements to support eye

health and improve vision. Dosage: take 160 mg of bilberry supplements twice daily.

45. Amenorrhea & absent periods = take chasteberry, make a tea from dried chasteberry or consume chasteberry supplements to help regulate menstrual cycles. Dosage: drink 1 cup of chasteberry tea 2-3 times daily or take 20-40 mg of chasteberry supplements daily.

46. Amenorrhea & irregular menstrual cycles = take chasteberry, consume chasteberry supplements or make a tea from dried chasteberry to help regulate menstrual cycles. Dosage: drink 1 cup of chasteberry tea 1-2 times daily or take 400-500 mg of chasteberry supplements daily.

47. Amnesia = take ginkgo biloba, make a tea from dried ginkgo biloba leaves or consume ginkgo biloba supplements to potentially benefit cognitive function and help manage amnesia. Dosage: drink 1 cup of ginkgo biloba tea 2-3 times daily or take 120-240 mg of ginkgo biloba supplements daily.

48. Amyloidosis = use turmeric, take turmeric supplements to reduce inflammation and support overall health. Dosage: take 400-600 mg of turmeric supplements 3 times daily.

49. Anal cancer = take green tea, drink green tea to support immune function and overall health during treatment. Dosage: drink 1 cup of green tea 2-3 times daily.

50. Anal fissure = use calendula, apply calendula ointment topically to promote healing and reduce pain. Dosage: apply calendula ointment 2-3 times daily.

51. Anal fistula = take turmeric, apply turmeric paste topically and consume turmeric supplements to reduce inflammation and support healing. Dosage: apply turmeric paste 2-3 times daily and take 400-600 mg of turmeric supplements 3 times daily.

52. Anal pain = use witch hazel, apply witch hazel topically to soothe and reduce anal pain. Dosage: apply witch hazel 2-3 times daily.

53. Anaphylaxis (post-recovery support) = take astragalus, consume astragalus supplements to support immune function. Dosage: take 500-1,000 mg of astragalus supplements 2-3 times daily.

54. Androgen insensitivity syndrome = use spearmint, drink spearmint tea to help balance hormone levels. Dosage: drink 1 cup of spearmint tea 2-3 times daily.

55. Anemia = take nettle, make a tea from dried nettle leaves or consume nettle supplements to help manage anemia. Dosage: drink 1 cup of nettle tea 2-3 times daily or take 300-600 mg of nettle supplements daily.

56. Anemia & iron deficiency = take nettle, make a tea from dried nettle leaves or consume nettle supplements to help increase iron levels and manage anemia. Dosage: drink 1 cup of nettle tea 2-3 times daily or take 300-600 mg of nettle supplements daily.

57. Angelman syndrome = use melatonin, take melatonin supplements to help regulate sleep patterns. Dosage: take 1-3 mg of melatonin supplements 30 minutes before bedtime.

58. Angina = take hawthorn, consume hawthorn supplements to support heart health and improve circulation. Dosage: take 160-900 mg of hawthorn supplements daily.

59. Angina & chest pain = take hawthorn, make a tea from dried hawthorn berries or consume hawthorn supplements to help manage angina and chest pain. Dosage: drink 1 cup of hawthorn tea 2-3 times daily or take 160-900 mg of hawthorn supplements daily.

60. Angioedema = use quercetin, take quercetin supplements to help reduce inflammation and support immune function. Dosage: take 500 mg of quercetin supplements twice daily.

61. Angiography (post-procedure support) = use ginger, drink ginger tea to reduce nausea and support circulation. Dosage: drink 1 cup of ginger tea 2-3 times daily.

62. Angioplasty (post-procedure support) = take garlic, consume garlic supplements to

support cardiovascular health and circulation. Dosage: take 600-1,200 mg of garlic supplements daily.

63. Animal and human bites = use echinacea, apply echinacea ointment topically to promote wound healing and prevent infection. Dosage: apply echinacea ointment 2-3 times daily.

64. Ankle pain = use arnica, apply arnica gel or cream topically to reduce pain and inflammation. Dosage: apply arnica gel or cream 2-3 times daily.

65. Ankylosing spondylitis = take turmeric, consume turmeric supplements or tea to reduce inflammation and alleviate symptoms. Dosage: take 400-600 mg of turmeric supplements 3 times daily or drink 1 cup of turmeric tea 2-3 times daily.

66. Ankylosing spondylitis & spinal arthritis = take turmeric, use turmeric powder in cooking or make a tea with turmeric and black pepper for anti-inflammatory effects to help manage ankylosing spondylitis. Dosage: take 400-600 mg of turmeric supplements 3 times daily or add

1 teaspoon of turmeric powder with a pinch of black pepper to meals daily.

67. Anorexia & appetite loss = take fennel, chew fennel seeds or make a tea from dried fennel seeds to help stimulate appetite and manage anorexia. Dosage: chew 1 teaspoon of fennel seeds or drink 1 cup of fennel tea 2-3 times daily.

68. Anorexia nervosa = use ginger, drink ginger tea to stimulate appetite and aid digestion. Dosage: drink 1 cup of ginger tea 2-3 times daily.

69. Anosmia = use rosemary, inhale rosemary essential oil or drink rosemary tea to potentially improve sense of smell. Dosage: inhale rosemary essential oil for 15-20 minutes or drink 1 cup of rosemary tea 2-3 times daily.

70. Antioxidant support & oxidative stress = take green tea, drink green tea regularly to provide antioxidant support and help reduce oxidative stress. Dosage: drink 1 cup of green tea 2-3 times daily.

71. Anxiety = take lavender, use essential oil in aromatherapy or make a tea from dried

flowers for anxiety relief. Dosage: inhale lavender essential oil for 15-20 minutes or drink 1 cup of lavender tea 2-3 times daily.

72. Anxiety and sleep = take passionflower, steep leaves and flowers in hot water for 10 minutes to make a tea for reducing anxiety and aiding sleep. Dosage: drink 1 cup of passionflower tea 30 minutes before bedtime.

73. Aortic aneurysm & aortic dissection = take garlic, consume raw garlic or garlic supplements to support cardiovascular health and help manage aortic aneurysm. Dosage: take 600-1,200 mg of garlic supplements daily or consume 1-2 cloves of raw garlic daily.

74. Aphasia & speech disorders = take ginkgo biloba, make a tea from dried ginkgo biloba leaves or consume ginkgo biloba supplements to potentially benefit cognitive function and manage aphasia. Dosage: drink 1 cup of ginkgo biloba tea 2-3 times daily or take 120-240 mg of ginkgo biloba supplements daily.

75. Aplastic anemia = consume dandelion root to support bone marrow health. Dosage: drink 1 cup of dandelion root tea 2-3 times daily or take 1-2 grams of dandelion root powder per day.

76. Appendicitis & abdominal pain = take ginger, chew raw ginger or make a tea from fresh ginger to help manage symptoms of appendicitis and abdominal pain. Dosage: chew a small piece of raw ginger 2-3 times daily or drink 1 cup of ginger tea 2-3 times daily.

77. Arrhythmia & irregular heartbeat = take hawthorn, make a tea from dried hawthorn berries or consume hawthorn supplements to help manage arrhythmia and irregular heartbeat. Dosage: drink 1 cup of hawthorn tea 2-3 times daily or take 160-900 mg of hawthorn supplements daily.

78. Arthritis = take turmeric, use turmeric powder in cooking or make a tea with turmeric and black pepper for anti-inflammatory effects. Dosage: take 400-600 mg of turmeric supplements 3 times

daily or add 1 teaspoon of turmeric powder with a pinch of black pepper to meals daily.

79. Arthritis & joint pain = take ginger, use ginger in cooking or make a tea from fresh ginger to help manage arthritis and joint pain. Dosage: add 1-2 teaspoons of fresh ginger to meals daily or drink 1 cup of ginger tea 2-3 times daily.

80. Arthropathy & joint diseases = take turmeric, use turmeric powder in cooking or make a tea with turmeric and black pepper for anti-inflammatory effects to help manage arthropathy. Dosage: take 400-600 mg of turmeric supplements 3 times daily or add 1 teaspoon of turmeric powder with a pinch of black pepper to meals daily.

81. Asbestosis & lung fibrosis = take mullein, make a tea from dried mullein leaves or consume mullein supplements to support lung health and help manage asbestosis. Dosage: drink 1 cup of mullein tea 2-3 times daily or take 300-500 mg of mullein supplements daily.

82. Asthma = take mullein, steep dried leaves in hot water for 10 minutes to make a tea to ease asthma symptoms. Dosage: drink 1 cup of mullein tea 2-3 times daily.

83. Asthma & bronchial spasms = take eucalyptus, use eucalyptus oil in steam inhalation or make a tea from dried eucalyptus leaves to help manage asthma. Dosage: inhale eucalyptus steam for 5-10 minutes 2-3 times daily or drink 1 cup of eucalyptus tea 2-3 times daily.

84. Atherosclerosis = take garlic, consume raw garlic or garlic supplements to potentially benefit cardiovascular health and help manage atherosclerosis. Dosage: take 600-1,200 mg of garlic supplements daily or consume 1-2 cloves of raw garlic daily.

85. Atherosclerosis & arterial plaque = take garlic, consume raw garlic or garlic supplements to help reduce arterial plaque and manage atherosclerosis. Dosage: take 600-1,200 mg of garlic supplements daily or consume 1-2 cloves of raw garlic daily.

86. Athlete's foot = take tea tree oil, apply diluted tea tree oil directly to affected areas to help manage athlete's foot. Dosage: apply 5% diluted tea tree oil 2-3 times daily.

87. Atopic dermatitis & eczema = take chamomile, apply chamomile-infused lotion or make a tea from dried chamomile flowers to help manage atopic dermatitis. Dosage: apply chamomile lotion 2-3 times daily or drink 1 cup of chamomile tea 2-3 times daily.

88. Attention deficit disorder (add) & hyperactivity = take ginkgo biloba, make a tea from dried ginkgo biloba leaves or consume ginkgo biloba supplements to help manage add and hyperactivity. Dosage: drink 1 cup of ginkgo biloba tea 2-3 times daily or take 120-240 mg of ginkgo biloba supplements daily.

89. Autoimmune hepatitis & liver inflammation = take milk thistle, consume milk thistle supplements to support liver health and help manage autoimmune hepatitis. Dosage: take 200-400 mg of milk thistle supplements 2-3 times daily.

90. Back pain = take willow bark, steep dried bark in hot water for 10-15 minutes to make a tea for back pain relief. Dosage: drink 1 cup of willow bark tea 2-3 times daily.

91. Back pain & sciatica = take devil's claw, consume devil's claw supplements or make a tea from dried devil's claw root to help manage back pain and sciatica. Dosage: drink 1 cup of devil's claw tea 2-3 times daily or take 600-1,200 mg of devil's claw supplements daily.

92. Bacterial vaginosis = use tea tree oil, apply diluted tea tree oil topically to help balance vaginal flora. Dosage: apply diluted tea tree oil to affected areas 2-3 times daily.

93. Bacterial vaginosis & vaginal infections = take tea tree oil, apply diluted tea tree oil topically to help manage bacterial vaginosis. Dosage: apply diluted tea tree oil to affected areas 2-3 times daily.

94. Bad breath = use parsley, chew fresh parsley leaves to naturally freshen breath. Dosage: chew a few fresh parsley leaves after meals as needed.

95. Baker's cyst = use ginger, apply ginger compresses or drink ginger tea to reduce swelling and pain. Dosage: apply ginger compresses 2-3 times daily or drink 1 cup of ginger tea 2-3 times daily.

96. Balanitis = use calendula, apply calendula cream or ointment topically to soothe and heal irritated skin. Dosage: apply calendula cream or ointment 2-3 times daily.

97. Barium enema (post-procedure support) = use chamomile, drink chamomile tea to calm the digestive system and reduce discomfort. Dosage: drink 1 cup of chamomile tea 2-3 times daily.

98. Barrett's esophagus & esophageal erosion = take slippery elm, make a tea from dried slippery elm bark or consume slippery elm supplements to help soothe esophageal erosion. Dosage: drink 1 cup of slippery elm tea 2-3 times daily or take 400-500 mg of slippery elm supplements daily.

99. Bartholin's cyst = use witch hazel, apply witch hazel compresses to the affected area to reduce inflammation and discomfort. Dosage: apply witch hazel compresses to the affected area 2-3 times daily.

100. Bedsores = take calendula, apply calendula cream or ointment to bedsores to help promote healing. Dosage: apply calendula cream or ointment to bedsores 2-3 times daily.

101. Bedsores & pressure ulcers = take aloe vera, apply fresh aloe vera gel directly to bedsores to help promote healing. Dosage: apply aloe vera gel to the affected areas 2-3 times daily.

102. Bedwetting (enuresis) = take corn silk, make a tea from dried corn silk to help manage bedwetting. Dosage: drink 1 cup of corn silk tea 2-3 times daily.

103. Bell's palsy & facial paralysis = take st. John's wort, make a tea from dried st. John's wort flowers or use st. John's wort

oil topically to help manage bell's palsy. Dosage: drink 1 cup of st. John's wort tea 2-3 times daily or apply st. John's wort oil to affected areas 2-3 times daily.

104. Benign prostatic hyperplasia (bph) & prostate enlargement = take saw palmetto, consume saw palmetto supplements to help manage symptoms of bph. Dosage: take 320 mg of saw palmetto supplements daily.

105. Biliary cirrhosis & liver damage = take milk thistle, consume milk thistle supplements to support liver health and help manage biliary cirrhosis. Dosage: take 200-400 mg of milk thistle supplements 2-3 times daily.

106. Biopsy (post-procedure support) = use chamomile, drink chamomile tea to promote relaxation and aid in recovery. Dosage: drink 1 cup of chamomile tea 2-3 times daily.

107. Bipolar disorder = take st. John's wort, make a tea from dried st. John's wort flowers or use st. John's wort oil topically to help manage symptoms of bipolar disorder. Dosage: drink 1 cup of st. John's wort tea 2-3 times daily or take 300-600 mg of st. John's wort supplements 3 times daily.

108. Bird flu = use elderberry, consume elderberry syrup or supplements to support the immune system during flu-like illnesses. Dosage: take 1 tablespoon of elderberry syrup 2-3 times daily or 500 mg of elderberry supplements daily.

109. Black eye = use arnica, apply arnica gel or cream topically to reduce bruising and inflammation. Dosage: apply arnica gel or cream to the affected area 2-3 times daily.

110. Bladder cancer = use green tea, drink green tea regularly to potentially support overall health and provide antioxidants. Dosage: drink 1-2 cups of green tea daily.

111. Bladder infection & cystitis = take cranberry, drink cranberry juice or consume dried cranberries to help manage bladder infections. Dosage: drink 1-2 cups of cranberry juice daily or consume 1/4 cup of dried cranberries daily.

112. Bladder pain syndrome (interstitial cystitis) = use marshmallow root, drink marshmallow root tea to soothe and support urinary tract health. Dosage: drink 1 cup of marshmallow root tea 2-3 times daily.

113. Bladder stones = take dandelion root, consume dandelion root tea or supplements to potentially support kidney and urinary tract health. Dosage: drink 1 cup of dandelion root tea 2-3 times daily or take 500 mg of dandelion root supplements daily.

114. Bleeding after menopause = use red clover, drink red clover tea to potentially help balance hormones and support overall health. Dosage: drink 1 cup of red clover tea 2-3 times daily.

115. Bleeding and fever = take yarrow, steep leaves and flowers in hot water for 10 minutes to make a tea to stop bleeding and reduce fever. Dosage: drink 1 cup of yarrow tea 2-3 times daily.

116. Bleeding gums & gum disease = take myrrh, use myrrh mouthwash or apply myrrh oil topically to help manage bleeding gums. Dosage: rinse with myrrh mouthwash 2-3 times daily or apply myrrh oil to gums 2-3 times daily.

117. Blisters & skin irritation = take calendula, apply calendula cream or ointment to blisters to help promote healing. Dosage: apply calendula cream or ointment to blisters 2-3 times daily.

118. Bloating = take fennel, steep dried seeds in hot water for 10 minutes to make a tea to reduce bloating. Dosage: drink 1 cup of fennel tea 2-3 times daily.

119. Bloating & gas = take peppermint, make a tea from dried peppermint leaves or chew fresh peppermint leaves to help relieve bloating. Dosage: drink 1 cup of peppermint tea 2-3 times daily or chew a few fresh peppermint leaves after meals.

120. Blood clots = take ginger, use ginger in cooking or make a tea from fresh ginger to potentially help prevent blood clots. Dosage: drink 1 cup of ginger tea 2-3 times daily or incorporate ginger into your diet regularly.

121. Blood clots & deep vein thrombosis (dvt) = take ginger, consume ginger tea or supplements to help prevent blood clots. Dosage: drink 1 cup of ginger tea 2-3 times daily or take 1,000 mg of ginger supplements daily.

122. Blood pressure and cholesterol = take hibiscus, brew dried flowers in hot water for 10 minutes to make a tea for lowering blood pressure and cholesterol. Dosage: drink 1 cup of hibiscus tea 2-3 times daily.

123. Blood sugar levels = take cinnamon, add powdered cinnamon to food or beverages, or make a tea by simmering cinnamon sticks in water. Dosage: consume 1-2 grams of cinnamon daily.

124. Blurred vision = take bilberry, consume bilberry supplements or make a tea from dried bilberry leaves to help manage blurred vision. Dosage: drink 1 cup of bilberry tea 2-3 times daily or take 160-240 mg of bilberry supplements daily.

125. Boils = take tea tree oil, apply diluted tea tree oil directly to boils to help manage symptoms. Dosage: apply diluted tea tree oil to boils 2-3 times daily.

126. Boils & abscesses = take turmeric, make a paste with turmeric powder and apply it topically to boils to help reduce inflammation. Dosage: apply turmeric paste to affected areas 2-3 times daily.

127. Bone cancer = use turmeric, consume turmeric supplements to potentially help reduce inflammation and support overall health. Dosage: take 500-2,000 mg of turmeric supplements daily.

128. Bone cyst = use boswellia, take boswellia supplements to potentially help reduce inflammation and support joint health. Dosage: take 300-500 mg of boswellia supplements 2-3 times daily.

129. Bone density = use horsetail, drink horsetail tea to potentially support bone health and density. Dosage: drink 1 cup of horsetail tea 2-3 times daily.

130. Bone health & osteoporosis = take horsetail, consume horsetail supplements or make a tea from dried horsetail to help support bone health. Dosage: drink 1 cup

of horsetail tea 2-3 times daily or take 300 mg of horsetail supplements daily.

131. Borderline personality disorder = use lavender, inhale lavender essential oil or drink lavender tea to potentially help reduce anxiety and promote relaxation. Dosage: inhale lavender essential oil as needed or drink 1 cup of lavender tea 2-3 times daily.

132. Botulism = use activated charcoal, take activated charcoal supplements to potentially help detoxify the body. Dosage: take 500-1,000 mg of activated charcoal supplements as needed, under medical supervision.

133. Bowel cancer = use garlic, consume raw garlic or garlic supplements to potentially support immune function and overall health. Dosage: consume 1-2 cloves of raw garlic daily or take 600-1,200 mg of garlic supplements daily.

134. Bowel incontinence = use pumpkin seed, consume pumpkin seed oil or seeds to potentially support urinary and bowel health. Dosage: take 1 tablespoon of pumpkin seed oil daily or consume a handful of pumpkin seeds daily.

135. Bowel polyps = use curcumin (from turmeric), take curcumin supplements to potentially help reduce inflammation and support gastrointestinal health. Dosage: take 500-1,000 mg of curcumin supplements daily.

136. Bowen's disease = use aloe vera, apply aloe vera gel topically to potentially help soothe and support skin health. Dosage: apply aloe vera gel to affected areas 2-3 times daily.

137. Braces and orthodontics (post-treatment care) = use chamomile, drink chamomile tea to potentially help reduce inflammation and promote relaxation. Dosage: drink 1 cup of chamomile tea 2-3 times daily.

138. Brain aneurysm & cerebral health = take ginger, make a tea from fresh ginger to help support cerebral health. Dosage: drink 1 cup of ginger tea 2-3 times daily.

139. Brain fog = take ginkgo biloba, make a tea from dried ginkgo biloba leaves or

consume ginkgo biloba supplements to potentially improve cognitive function and manage brain fog. Dosage: drink 1 cup of ginkgo biloba tea 2-3 times daily or take 120-240 mg of ginkgo biloba supplements daily.

140. Breast pain & mastalgia = take evening primrose oil, consume evening primrose oil supplements to help manage breast pain. Dosage: take 1,000 mg of evening primrose oil supplements 2-3 times daily.

141. Breast tenderness = take chasteberry (vitex), consume chasteberry supplements or make a tea from dried chasteberry fruit to help manage breast tenderness. Dosage: drink 1 cup of chasteberry tea 2-3 times daily or take 400-500 mg of chasteberry supplements daily.

142. Breastfeeding problems = take fenugreek, consume fenugreek seeds or supplements to help support milk production and manage breastfeeding problems. Dosage: take 1-2 grams of fenugreek seeds 3 times daily or 600-1,200 mg of fenugreek supplements daily.

143. Bronchiolitis = use mullein, drink mullein tea to soothe the respiratory tract and reduce inflammation. Dosage: drink 1 cup of mullein tea 2-3 times daily.

144. Bronchitis = take eucalyptus, use eucalyptus oil in steam inhalation or make a tea from dried eucalyptus leaves to help manage bronchitis symptoms. Dosage: inhale eucalyptus steam for 5-10 minutes 2-3 times daily or drink 1 cup of eucalyptus tea 2-3 times daily.

145. Bronchitis & respiratory infections = take thyme, make a tea from dried thyme leaves or use thyme essential oil in steam inhalation to help manage bronchitis. Dosage: drink 1 cup of thyme tea 2-3 times daily or inhale thyme steam for 5-10 minutes 2-3 times daily.

146. Bronchodilators (natural support) = use lobelia, take lobelia supplements to help relax the airways and ease breathing. Dosage: take 0.5-1 ml of lobelia tincture 3 times daily.

147. Brown recluse spider bite & skin infection = take calendula, apply calendula

ointment to the affected area to help soothe skin infections. Dosage: apply calendula ointment to affected areas 2-3 times daily.

148. Brucellosis = use garlic, consume raw garlic or garlic supplements to support the immune system and fight bacterial infections. Dosage: consume 1-2 cloves of raw garlic daily or take 600-1,200 mg of garlic supplements daily.

149. Brugada syndrome = use hawthorn, take hawthorn supplements to support heart health (under medical supervision). Dosage: take 160-900 mg of hawthorn extract daily.

150. Bruises = take arnica, apply arnica cream or gel to bruises for faster healing. Dosage: apply arnica cream or gel to bruises 2-3 times daily.

151. Bruxism = use chamomile, drink chamomile tea before bed to reduce stress and promote relaxation. Dosage: drink 1 cup of chamomile tea 30 minutes before bed.

152. Bruxism & teeth grinding = take valerian root, consume valerian root supplements or make a tea from dried valerian root to help relax muscles. Dosage: drink 1 cup of valerian root tea 30 minutes before bed or take 400-900 mg of valerian root supplements daily.

153. Budd-Chiari syndrome = take milk thistle to support liver function. Dosage: take 150-300 mg of milk thistle extract 2-3 times daily.

154. Bulging eyes (exophthalmos) = use bilberry, consume bilberry supplements to support eye health. Dosage: take 160-240 mg of bilberry extract daily.

155. Bulimia = use ginger, drink ginger tea to soothe the digestive system and help manage nausea. Dosage: drink 1 cup of ginger tea 2-3 times daily.

156. Bulimia nervosa & eating disorder = take licorice root, make a tea from dried licorice root to help support digestive health. Dosage: drink 1 cup of licorice root tea 2-3 times daily.

157. Bullous pemphigoid = use aloe vera, apply aloe vera gel topically to soothe and heal the skin. Dosage: apply aloe vera gel to affected areas 2-3 times daily.

158. Bunions = use turmeric, apply turmeric paste topically to reduce inflammation and pain. Dosage: apply turmeric paste to bunions 2-3 times daily.

159. Bunions & foot pain = take turmeric, make a paste with turmeric powder and apply it topically to bunions to help reduce inflammation. Dosage: apply turmeric paste to bunions 2-3 times daily.

160. Burns = take aloe vera, apply fresh aloe vera gel directly to burns to help soothe and promote healing. Dosage: apply aloe vera gel to burns as needed throughout the day.

161. Burns and scalds = use aloe vera, apply aloe vera gel topically to soothe and promote healing of burns. Dosage: apply aloe vera gel to burns as needed throughout the day.

162. Burns and skin irritations = take aloe vera, cut a leaf and extract the gel. Apply directly to burns or skin irritations. Dosage: apply aloe vera gel to burns or skin irritations as needed throughout the day.

163. Bursitis = use ginger, drink ginger tea to reduce inflammation and alleviate pain. Dosage: drink 1 cup of ginger tea 2-3 times daily.

164. Bursitis & joint inflammation = take devil's claw, consume devil's claw supplements or make a tea from dried devil's claw root to help manage bursitis. Dosage: drink 1 cup of devil's claw tea 2-3 times daily or take 600-1,200 mg of devil's claw supplements daily.

165. Cachexia & muscle wasting = take ashwagandha, consume ashwagandha supplements to help support muscle health. Dosage: take 300-500 mg of ashwagandha supplements 2-3 times daily.

166. Calcaneal spur & heel pain = take turmeric, use turmeric powder in cooking or make a tea with turmeric and black pepper to help manage heel pain. Dosage:

drink 1 cup of turmeric tea 2-3 times daily or consume 500-2,000 mg of turmeric supplements daily.

167. Candida = take oregano oil, dilute and take internally or apply topically to combat candida infections. Dosage: take 2-4 drops of oregano oil in a glass of water 2-3 times daily, or apply diluted oregano oil topically as needed.

168. Candida overgrowth & fungal infection = take oregano oil, use oregano oil capsules or diluted oregano oil to help manage candida overgrowth. Dosage: take 200-600 mg of oregano oil capsules daily or apply diluted oregano oil topically 2-3 times daily.

169. Canker sores = take licorice root, use a licorice root mouthwash to help heal canker sores. Dosage: use licorice root mouthwash 2-3 times daily.

170. Canker sores & mouth ulcers = take licorice, make a tea from dried licorice root or use licorice extract as a mouthwash to help soothe canker sores.

Dosage: use licorice root mouthwash 2-3 times daily.

171. Carcinoid syndrome & neuroendocrine tumors = take milk thistle, make a tea from dried milk thistle or consume milk thistle supplements to help support liver health. Dosage: drink 1 cup of milk thistle tea 2-3 times daily or take 150-450 mg of milk thistle supplements daily.

172. Cardiomyopathy = take astragalus to improve heart function. Dosage: drink 1-2 cups of astragalus tea daily or take 500-1,000 mg of astragalus extract twice daily.

173. Carpal tunnel syndrome = take turmeric, use turmeric powder in cooking or make a tea with turmeric and black pepper for anti-inflammatory effects to help manage carpal tunnel syndrome. Dosage: drink 1 cup of turmeric tea 2-3 times daily or take 500-2,000 mg of turmeric supplements daily.

174. Carpal tunnel syndrome & wrist pain = take turmeric, consume turmeric supplements or make a tea with turmeric and black pepper to help reduce

inflammation. Dosage: take 500-2,000 mg of turmeric supplements daily or drink 1 cup of turmeric tea 2-3 times daily.

175. Cat scratch fever & bacterial infection = take echinacea, make a tea from dried echinacea or consume echinacea supplements to help support the immune system. Dosage: drink 1 cup of echinacea tea 2-3 times daily or take 300 mg of echinacea supplements 3 times daily.

176. Cataracts = take bilberry, consume bilberry supplements or make a tea from dried bilberry leaves to support eye health and potentially benefit cataracts. Dosage: take 160-240 mg of bilberry extract daily.

177. Cataracts & vision impairment = take bilberry, consume bilberry supplements or make a tea from dried bilberry leaves to help support eye health. Dosage: take 160-240 mg of bilberry extract daily or drink 1 cup of bilberry tea 2-3 times daily.

178. Cavernoma = use turmeric, consume turmeric supplements to potentially help reduce inflammation and support overall

health. Dosage: take 500-2,000 mg of turmeric supplements daily.

179. Cavernous sinus thrombosis = use ginger, drink ginger tea to potentially help improve circulation and reduce inflammation. Dosage: drink 1 cup of ginger tea 2-3 times daily.

180. Celiac disease = take chamomile, make a tea from dried chamomile flowers to help soothe gastrointestinal symptoms in celiac disease. Dosage: drink 1 cup of chamomile tea 2-3 times daily.

181. Celiac disease & gluten sensitivity = take chamomile, make a tea from dried chamomile flowers to help support digestive health. Dosage: drink 1 cup of chamomile tea 2-3 times daily.

182. Cellulite = take gotu kola, apply gotu kola cream to affected areas to reduce cellulite. Dosage: apply gotu kola cream to affected areas 2-3 times daily.

183. Cellulitis = use garlic, consume raw garlic or garlic supplements to help fight bacterial infections and support the immune system. Dosage: consume 1-2

cloves of raw garlic daily or take 600-1,200 mg of garlic supplements daily.

184. Cellulitis & skin infections = take echinacea, consume echinacea supplements or make a tea from dried echinacea to help boost the immune system. Dosage: take 300 mg of echinacea supplements 3 times daily or drink 1 cup of echinacea tea 2-3 times daily.

185. Central sleep apnea & breathing disorders = take valerian root, consume valerian root supplements or make a tea from dried valerian root to help manage sleep apnea. Dosage: drink 1 cup of valerian root tea 30 minutes before bed or take 400-900 mg of valerian root supplements daily.

186. Cerebral palsy = use ginkgo biloba, take ginkgo biloba supplements to potentially help improve circulation and support brain health. Dosage: take 120-240 mg of ginkgo biloba supplements daily.

187. Cerebral palsy & muscle spasticity = take chamomile, make a tea from dried chamomile flowers or use chamomile

essential oil in a bath to help relax muscles. Dosage: drink 1 cup of chamomile tea 2-3 times daily or add a few drops of chamomile essential oil to a warm bath.

188. Cerebral palsy & neurological disorder = take ginkgo biloba, make a tea from dried ginkgo biloba leaves or consume ginkgo biloba supplements to help support neurological health. Dosage: drink 1 cup of ginkgo biloba tea 2-3 times daily or take 120-240 mg of ginkgo biloba supplements daily.

189. Cervical cancer = use green tea, drink green tea regularly to potentially provide antioxidants and support overall health. Dosage: drink 2-3 cups of green tea daily.

190. Cervical dysplasia & abnormal pap smear = take green tea, drink green tea regularly to provide antioxidant support and potentially manage cervical dysplasia. Dosage: drink 2-3 cups of green tea daily.

191. Cervical spondylosis = use turmeric, consume turmeric supplements or tea to help reduce inflammation and alleviate

pain. Dosage: drink 1 cup of turmeric tea 2-3 times daily or take 500-2,000 mg of turmeric supplements daily.

192. Chagas disease = use pau d'arco for its antimicrobial properties. Dosage: drink 1 cup of pau d'arco tea 2-3 times daily or take 500-1,000 mg of pau d'arco supplements daily.

193. Chagas disease & parasitic infection = take garlic, consume raw garlic or garlic supplements to help manage parasitic infections. Dosage: consume 1-2 cloves of raw garlic daily or take 600-1,200 mg of garlic supplements daily.

194. Charcot-marie-tooth disease = use evening primrose oil, take evening primrose oil supplements to potentially help improve nerve health and reduce symptoms. Dosage: take 500-1,000 mg of evening primrose oil supplements 2-3 times daily.

195. Charles bonnet syndrome = use bilberry, consume bilberry supplements to support eye health and potentially improve vision.

Dosage: take 160-240 mg of bilberry extract daily.

196. Cheilitis & cracked lips = take coconut oil, apply coconut oil directly to cracked lips to help moisturize and heal. Dosage: apply coconut oil to lips as needed.

197. Chemical burns & skin injury = take aloe vera, apply aloe vera gel to the affected area to help soothe chemical burns. Dosage: apply aloe vera gel to affected areas as needed throughout the day.

198. Chemotherapy (support during treatment) = use ginger, drink ginger tea to help reduce nausea and support digestion. Dosage: drink 1 cup of ginger tea 2-3 times daily.

199. Chest infection = use thyme, drink thyme tea to help clear mucus and support respiratory health. Dosage: drink 1 cup of thyme tea 2-3 times daily.

200. Chickenpox = use calendula, apply calendula lotion or cream topically to soothe itchy skin and promote healing. Dosage: apply calendula lotion or cream to affected areas 2-3 times daily.

201. Chikungunya virus & mosquito-borne illness = take ginger, make a tea from fresh ginger to help manage symptoms of chikungunya virus. Dosage: drink 1 cup of ginger tea 2-3 times daily.

202. Chilblains = use ginger, drink ginger tea to improve circulation and reduce inflammation. Dosage: drink 1 cup of ginger tea 2-3 times daily.

203. Chilblains & cold injury = take cayenne pepper, apply cayenne pepper cream to the affected areas to help improve circulation. Dosage: apply cayenne pepper cream to affected areas 2-3 times daily.

204. Chilblains & cold-induced swelling = take ginger, make a tea from fresh ginger slices or use ginger essential oil in a warm compress to help manage chilblains. Dosage: drink 1 cup of ginger tea 2-3 times daily or apply a warm compress with a few drops of ginger essential oil to the affected area.

205. Childhood cataracts = use bilberry, consume bilberry supplements to support eye health and potentially improve vision. Dosage: take 160-240 mg of bilberry extract daily.

206. Children's flu = use elderberry, give elderberry syrup to support the immune system and reduce flu symptoms. Dosage: give 1-2 teaspoons of elderberry syrup 2-3 times daily for children.

207. Chiropractic (post-treatment support) = use arnica, apply arnica gel or cream topically to reduce muscle pain and inflammation. Dosage: apply arnica gel or cream to affected areas 2-3 times daily.

208. Chlamydia = use echinacea, consume echinacea tea or supplements to support the immune system and fight infection. Dosage: drink 1 cup of echinacea tea 2-3 times daily or take 300 mg of echinacea supplements 3 times daily.

209. Chlamydia & bacterial infections = take goldenseal, consume goldenseal supplements or make a tea from dried goldenseal to help manage bacterial infections. Dosage: take 250-500 mg of goldenseal supplements 3 times daily or

drink 1 cup of goldenseal tea 2-3 times daily.

210. Cholecystitis & gallbladder inflammation = take dandelion root, make a tea from dried dandelion root to help support gallbladder health. Dosage: drink 1 cup of dandelion root tea 2-3 times daily.

211. Cholecystitis (acute) = use dandelion root, drink dandelion root tea to support liver and gallbladder health. Dosage: drink 1 cup of dandelion root tea 2-3 times daily.

212. Cholera = use goldenseal, take goldenseal supplements to support the immune system and fight bacterial infections. Dosage: take 250-500 mg of goldenseal supplements 3 times daily.

213. Chronic fatigue syndrome & exhaustion = take ashwagandha, consume ashwagandha supplements or make a tea from dried ashwagandha root to help manage chronic fatigue. Dosage: take 300-500 mg of ashwagandha supplements 2-3 times daily or drink 1 cup of ashwagandha tea 2-3 times daily.

214. Chronic fatigue syndrome & persistent exhaustion = take siberian ginseng, consume siberian ginseng supplements to help support energy levels. Dosage: take 100-200 mg of siberian ginseng supplements 2-3 times daily.

215. Chronic laryngitis & voice box inflammation = take licorice root, make a tea from dried licorice root to help soothe the throat. Dosage: drink 1 cup of licorice root tea 2-3 times daily.

216. Chronic obstructive pulmonary disease (COPD) = use mullein to help clear mucus and improve lung function. Dosage: drink 1-2 cups of mullein tea daily or take 300-500 mg of mullein supplements 2-3 times daily.

217. Chronic obstructive pulmonary disease (copd) & breathing difficulties = take mullein, make a tea from dried mullein leaves or consume mullein supplements to support respiratory health. Dosage: drink 1 cup of mullein tea 2-3 times daily or take 300-500 mg of mullein supplements 2-3 times daily.

218. Cirrhosis = use milk thistle for liver support and detoxification. Dosage: take 200-400 mg of silymarin (active compound in milk thistle) supplements 2-3 times daily.

219. Cirrhosis & liver scarring = take milk thistle, consume milk thistle supplements to support liver health and help manage cirrhosis. Dosage: take 200-400 mg of milk thistle extract 2-3 times daily.

220. Claustrophobia = use valerian root, take valerian root supplements or drink valerian tea to reduce anxiety and promote relaxation. Dosage: take 400-900 mg of valerian root extract 2 hours before bedtime or drink 1 cup of valerian tea 2-3 times daily.

221. Cleft lip and palate (post-surgery support) = use chamomile, drink chamomile tea to reduce inflammation and promote healing. Dosage: drink 1 cup of chamomile tea 2-3 times daily.

222. Clostridium difficile (c. Diff) infection = use oregano oil, take oregano oil supplements to help fight bacterial infections and support gut health. Dosage: take 200 mg of oregano oil supplements 2-3 times daily.

223. Cluster headaches & severe headaches = take feverfew, make a tea from dried feverfew leaves or consume feverfew supplements to help manage cluster headaches. Dosage: drink 1 cup of feverfew tea 2-3 times daily or take 100-300 mg of feverfew supplements daily.

224. Cognitive function and skin health = take gotu kola, brew leaves in hot water for 10 minutes to make a tea for enhancing cognitive function and skin health. Dosage: drink 1 cup of gotu kola tea 2-3 times daily.

225. Cold sores = take lemon balm, apply lemon balm cream or ointment to cold sores to help manage symptoms. Dosage: apply lemon balm cream or ointment to cold sores 2-3 times daily.

226. Cold sores & herpes simplex = take lemon balm, apply lemon balm ointment to cold sores or make a tea from dried lemon balm leaves to help manage herpes

simplex. Dosage: apply lemon balm ointment to cold sores 2-3 times daily or drink 1 cup of lemon balm tea 2-3 times daily.

227. Colic = take chamomile, steep dried flowers in hot water for 10 minutes to make a tea to soothe colic in infants. Dosage: give 1-2 ounces of cooled chamomile tea to infants 2-3 times daily.

228. Colic & abdominal pain in infants = take fennel, make a tea from dried fennel seeds or use fennel essential oil in a warm compress to help soothe colic. Dosage: give 1-2 ounces of cooled fennel tea to infants 2-3 times daily.

229. Colitis = take marshmallow root, steep dried root in hot water for 10 minutes to make a tea to soothe colitis symptoms. Dosage: drink 1 cup of marshmallow root tea 2-3 times daily.

230. Colitis & inflammatory bowel disease (ibd) = take slippery elm, make a tea from dried slippery elm bark or consume slippery elm supplements to help soothe the digestive tract. Dosage: drink 1 cup of slippery elm tea 2-3 times daily or take 400-500 mg of slippery elm supplements 2-3 times daily.

231. Common cold = take echinacea, consume echinacea supplements or make a tea from dried echinacea roots to help manage common cold symptoms. Dosage: drink 1 cup of echinacea tea 2-3 times daily or take 300 mg of echinacea supplements 3 times daily.

232. Complex regional pain syndrome (CRPS) = consume devil's claw for pain relief. Dosage: take 500-1,000 mg of devil's claw extract 2-3 times daily.

233. Concussion & head injury = take arnica, apply arnica cream to the affected area to help reduce swelling and pain. Dosage: apply arnica cream to affected areas 2-3 times daily.

234. Congestive heart failure = take coenzyme Q10 to support heart function. Dosage: take 100-200 mg of coenzyme Q10 supplements daily.

235. Conjunctivitis = take chamomile, make a tea from dried chamomile flowers or use

chamomile-infused eye drops to help manage conjunctivitis. Dosage: use cooled chamomile tea as an eye wash 2-3 times daily.

236. Conjunctivitis & eye infection = take chamomile, make a tea from dried chamomile flowers and use as an eye wash to help manage conjunctivitis. Dosage: use cooled chamomile tea as an eye wash 2-3 times daily.

237. Conjunctivitis & pink eye = take chamomile, use chamomile-infused eye drops or make a tea from dried chamomile flowers to help manage conjunctivitis. Dosage: use chamomile eye drops as needed or use cooled chamomile tea as an eye wash 2-3 times daily.

238. Constipation = take senna, consume senna tea or supplements to help relieve constipation. Dosage: drink 1 cup of senna tea before bed or take 17.2 mg of senna supplements once daily.

239. Constipation & irregular bowel movements = take psyllium husk, consume psyllium husk supplements or mix with water to help regulate bowel movements. Dosage: take 1-2 teaspoons of psyllium husk powder mixed in a glass of water 1-2 times daily.

240. Convulsions & seizures = take valerian root, consume valerian root supplements or make a tea from dried valerian root to help manage seizures. Dosage: take 400-900 mg of valerian root extract 2 hours before bedtime or drink 1 cup of valerian tea 2-3 times daily.

241. Corn & calluses = take calendula, apply calendula cream or ointment to corns and calluses to help soften and heal. Dosage: apply calendula cream or ointment to corns and calluses 2-3 times daily.

242. Corneal abrasion & eye injury = take eyebright, make a tea from dried eyebright herb or use eyebright eye drops to help soothe corneal abrasions. Dosage: use cooled eyebright tea as an eye wash 2-3 times daily or follow the instructions on eyebright eye drops.

243.Cough = take licorice root, steep dried root in hot water for 10 minutes to make a tea to soothe cough. Dosage: drink 1 cup of licorice root tea 2-3 times daily.

244.Coughs and digestive issues = take marshmallow root, boil root in water for 15 minutes to make a tea for soothing coughs and digestive issues. Dosage: drink 1 cup of marshmallow root tea 2-3 times daily.

245.Cramps & muscle spasms = take magnesium, consume magnesium-rich foods or supplements to help manage muscle cramps. Dosage: take 300-400 mg of magnesium supplements daily.

246.Crohn's disease & inflammatory bowel disease (ibd) = take turmeric, use turmeric powder in cooking or make a tea with turmeric and black pepper to help reduce inflammation. Dosage: take 500-2,000 mg of turmeric supplements daily or drink 1 cup of turmeric tea 2-3 times daily.

247.Croup & respiratory infections in children = take thyme, make a tea from dried thyme leaves or use thyme essential oil in steam inhalation to help manage croup. Dosage: drink 1 cup of thyme tea 2-3 times daily or add a few drops of thyme essential oil to a bowl of hot water for steam inhalation.

248.Cushing's syndrome & hypercortisolism = take reishi mushroom, consume reishi mushroom supplements to help support adrenal function. Dosage: take 500-1,000 mg of reishi mushroom supplements daily.

249.Cystic fibrosis = use eucalyptus to improve respiratory function. Dosage: drink 1-2 cups of eucalyptus tea daily or inhale eucalyptus steam for 10-15 minutes daily.

250.Cystic fibrosis & lung disease = take marshmallow root, make a tea from dried marshmallow root to help support respiratory health. Dosage: drink 1 cup of marshmallow root tea 2-3 times daily.

251.Cystic fibrosis & mucus build-up = take mullein, make a tea from dried mullein leaves or consume mullein supplements to help manage mucus build-up. Dosage:

drink 1 cup of mullein tea 2-3 times daily or take 300-500 mg of mullein supplements 2-3 times daily.

252. Cystitis = take cranberry, drink cranberry juice or consume dried cranberries to help manage cystitis. Dosage: drink 1-2 cups of cranberry juice daily or consume 1/4 to 1/2 cup of dried cranberries daily.

253. Cystitis & urinary tract infections (utis) = take cranberry, drink cranberry juice or consume dried cranberries to help manage cystitis. Dosage: drink 8-16 ounces of cranberry juice daily or consume 1/4-1/2 cup of dried cranberries daily.

254. Dandruff = take tea tree oil, use shampoo containing tea tree oil or add tea tree oil to your regular shampoo to help manage dandruff. Dosage: use tea tree oil shampoo 2-3 times weekly or add a few drops of tea tree oil to your regular shampoo.

255. Dandruff & scalp itching = take tea tree oil, use a shampoo with tea tree oil or apply diluted tea tree oil to the scalp to help manage dandruff. Dosage: use tea tree oil shampoo 2-3 times weekly or apply a few drops of diluted tea tree oil to the scalp daily.

256. Deep vein thrombosis (DVT) = consume ginger to improve blood circulation. Dosage: drink 1-2 cups of ginger tea daily or take 500-1,000 mg of ginger supplements 2-3 times daily.

257. Deep vein thrombosis (dvt) & blood clot = take ginger, make a tea from fresh ginger to help manage blood clotting. Dosage: drink 1 cup of ginger tea 2-3 times daily.

258. Degenerative disc disease & spinal degeneration = take turmeric, use turmeric powder in cooking or make a tea with turmeric and black pepper to help manage inflammation. Dosage: take 500-2,000 mg of turmeric supplements daily or drink 1 cup of turmeric tea 2-3 times daily.

259. Dehydration = take coconut water, drink coconut water to help rehydrate the body.

Dosage: drink 8-16 ounces of coconut water daily.

260. Dementia = take ginkgo biloba, make a tea from dried ginkgo biloba leaves or consume ginkgo biloba supplements to potentially benefit cognitive function in dementia. Dosage: drink 1 cup of ginkgo biloba tea 2-3 times daily or take 120-240 mg of ginkgo biloba supplements daily.

261. Dental abscess & tooth infection = take clove oil, apply clove oil to the affected tooth to help manage pain and infection. Dosage: apply 1-2 drops of clove oil to the affected tooth 2-3 times daily.

262. Depression = take st. John's wort, steep dried flowers in hot water for 10-15 minutes to make a tea for depression and mood swings. Dosage: drink 1 cup of st. John's wort tea 2-3 times daily or take 300-600 mg of st. John's wort supplements 2-3 times daily.

263. Dermatitis & skin irritation = take chamomile, apply chamomile-infused lotion or make a tea from dried chamomile flowers to help manage dermatitis. Dosage: apply chamomile lotion 2-3 times daily or drink 1 cup of chamomile tea 2-3 times daily.

264. Dermatomyositis = take cat's claw for its anti-inflammatory properties. Dosage: take 20-60 mg of cat's claw extract 2-3 times daily.

265. Diabetes = take fenugreek, soak seeds overnight in water and consume the water on an empty stomach to help regulate blood sugar levels. Dosage: soak 1-2 teaspoons of fenugreek seeds overnight and consume the water on an empty stomach daily.

266. Diabetic neuropathy = use alpha-lipoic acid to relieve nerve pain. Dosage: take 600-1,200 mg of alpha-lipoic acid supplements daily.

267. Diabetic neuropathy & nerve pain = take alpha-lipoic acid, consume alpha-lipoic acid supplements to help manage nerve pain in diabetic neuropathy. Dosage: take 600-1,200 mg of alpha-lipoic acid supplements daily.

268. Diaper rash = take calendula, apply calendula cream or ointment to affected areas to help soothe diaper rash. Dosage: apply calendula cream or ointment to the affected area 2-3 times daily.

269. Diarrhea = take blackberry leaf, steep dried leaves in hot water for 10 minutes to make a tea to relieve diarrhea. Dosage: drink 1 cup of blackberry leaf tea 2-3 times daily.

270. Diarrhea & gastroenteritis = take blackberry leaf, make a tea from dried blackberry leaves to help manage diarrhea. Dosage: drink 1 cup of blackberry leaf tea 2-3 times daily.

271. Digestion and lactation = take fenugreek, soak seeds in water overnight and drink the water or use the seeds in cooking for digestion and lactation. Dosage: drink 1 cup of fenugreek water daily or use 1-2 teaspoons of fenugreek seeds in cooking daily.

272. Digestive issues = take ginger, chew raw ginger or make a tea from fresh ginger slices to alleviate digestive problems. Dosage: chew a small piece of raw ginger 2-3 times daily or drink 1 cup of ginger tea 2-3 times daily.

273. Digestive issues and sore throats = take licorice root, boil roots in water for 10-15 minutes to make a tea for digestive issues and sore throats. Dosage: drink 1 cup of licorice root tea 2-3 times daily.

274. Diphtheria & bacterial infection = take garlic, consume raw garlic or garlic supplements to help manage diphtheria. Dosage: eat 2-3 raw garlic cloves daily or take 600-1,200 mg of garlic supplements daily.

275. Discoid lupus & skin condition = take turmeric, apply turmeric paste to affected skin areas to help manage discoid lupus. Dosage: apply turmeric paste to affected areas 1-2 times daily.

276. Diverticulitis = take slippery elm, consume slippery elm supplements or make a tea from dried slippery elm bark to help manage diverticulitis symptoms. Dosage: drink 1 cup of slippery elm tea 2-

3 times daily or take 400-500 mg of slippery elm supplements 2-3 times daily.

277. Diverticulitis & intestinal inflammation = take peppermint, make a tea from dried peppermint leaves to help manage diverticulitis. Dosage: drink 1 cup of peppermint tea 2-3 times daily.

278. Dizziness & vertigo = take ginger, chew raw ginger or make a tea from fresh ginger to help manage dizziness and vertigo. Dosage: chew a small piece of raw ginger 2-3 times daily or drink 1 cup of ginger tea 2-3 times daily.

279. Down syndrome = take green tea, consume green tea regularly to potentially benefit cognitive function in down syndrome. Dosage: drink 1-2 cups of green tea daily.

280. Drooling & excessive salivation = take sage, make a tea from dried sage leaves to help reduce drooling. Dosage: drink 1 cup of sage tea 2-3 times daily.

281. Drowsiness = take peppermint, inhale peppermint essential oil or make a tea from dried peppermint leaves to help alleviate drowsiness. Dosage: inhale peppermint essential oil as needed or drink 1 cup of peppermint tea 2-3 times daily.

282. Dry eyes & eye irritation = take bilberry, consume bilberry supplements or make a tea from dried bilberry leaves to support eye health. Dosage: take 160-240 mg of bilberry extract daily or drink 1 cup of bilberry tea 2-3 times daily.

283. Dry mouth & xerostomia = take marshmallow root, make a tea from dried marshmallow root or use marshmallow root lozenges to help manage dry mouth. Dosage: drink 1 cup of marshmallow root tea 2-3 times daily or use marshmallow root lozenges as needed.

284. Dry skin = take coconut oil, apply coconut oil topically to moisturize dry skin. Dosage: apply coconut oil to dry skin as needed.

285. Dysentery & intestinal infection = take goldenseal, make a tea from dried goldenseal root to help manage dysentery. Dosage: drink 1 cup of goldenseal tea 2-3

times daily or take 250-500 mg of goldenseal supplements 2-3 times daily.

286. Dysentery & severe diarrhea = take goldenseal, make a tea from dried goldenseal or consume goldenseal supplements to help manage dysentery. Dosage: drink 1 cup of goldenseal tea 2-3 times daily or take 250-500 mg of goldenseal supplements 2-3 times daily.

287. Dyslexia & learning disorder = take ginkgo biloba, make a tea from dried ginkgo biloba leaves or consume ginkgo biloba supplements to help support cognitive function. Dosage: drink 1 cup of ginkgo biloba tea 2-3 times daily or take 120-240 mg of ginkgo biloba supplements daily.

288. Dysmenorrhea & menstrual pain = take ginger, make a tea from fresh ginger to help manage dysmenorrhea. Dosage: drink 1 cup of ginger tea 2-3 times daily.

289. Dyspareunia & painful intercourse = take evening primrose oil, consume evening primrose oil supplements to help manage dyspareunia. Dosage: take 500-1,000 mg of evening primrose oil supplements daily.

290. Dyspepsia & indigestion = take peppermint, make a tea from dried peppermint leaves or chew fresh peppermint leaves to help manage indigestion. Dosage: drink 1 cup of peppermint tea 2-3 times daily or chew fresh peppermint leaves as needed.

291. Dysphagia & swallowing difficulty = take marshmallow root, make a tea from dried marshmallow root to help soothe the esophagus. Dosage: drink 1 cup of marshmallow root tea 2-3 times daily.

292. Dysphonia & voice disorder = take licorice root, make a tea from dried licorice root to help soothe the throat and manage dysphonia. Dosage: drink 1 cup of licorice root tea 2-3 times daily.

293. Dystonia & muscle contractions = take valerian root, consume valerian root supplements or make a tea from dried valerian root to help manage muscle contractions. Dosage: take 400-900 mg of valerian root extract 2 hours before

bedtime or drink 1 cup of valerian tea 2-3 times daily.

294. Ear infections & otitis = take garlic oil, apply warm garlic oil to the affected ear to help manage ear infections. Dosage: apply a few drops of warm garlic oil to the affected ear 2-3 times daily.

295. Earache & ear pain = take mullein, make a tea from dried mullein leaves and use as ear drops to help manage earache. Dosage: drink 1 cup of mullein tea 2-3 times daily or use a few drops of mullein oil in the affected ear daily.

296. Ebola virus & viral infection = take echinacea, make a tea from dried echinacea or consume echinacea supplements to help support the immune system. Dosage: drink 1 cup of echinacea tea 2-3 times daily or take 300-500 mg of echinacea supplements 2-3 times daily.

297. Echinococcosis & parasitic infection = take wormwood, make a tea from dried wormwood leaves to help manage echinococcosis. Dosage: drink 1 cup of wormwood tea 2-3 times daily.

298. Eclampsia & pregnancy complication = take ginger, make a tea from fresh ginger to help manage symptoms of eclampsia. Dosage: drink 1 cup of ginger tea 2-3 times daily.

299. Eczema = take calendula, apply calendula oil or cream to affected areas for eczema relief. Dosage: apply calendula oil or cream to the affected area 2-3 times daily.

300. Eczema & atopic dermatitis = take licorice root, apply licorice root cream or ointment to the affected areas to help manage eczema. Dosage: apply licorice root cream or ointment to the affected area 2-3 times daily.

301. Edema & fluid retention = take dandelion, make a tea from dried dandelion leaves or consume dandelion supplements to help manage edema. Dosage: drink 1 cup of dandelion tea 2-3 times daily or take 500-1,000 mg of dandelion supplements daily.

302. Edema & swelling = take dandelion, make a tea from dried dandelion leaves or consume dandelion supplements to help

reduce swelling. Dosage: drink 1 cup of dandelion tea 2-3 times daily or take 500-1,000 mg of dandelion supplements daily.

303. Ehlers-Danlos syndrome = consume collagen supplements to support connective tissue health. Dosage: take 2.5-15 grams of collagen peptides daily.

304. Ehlers-danlos syndrome & connective tissue disorder = take ginger, make a tea from fresh ginger to help manage symptoms of ehlers-danlos syndrome. Dosage: drink 1 cup of ginger tea 2-3 times daily.

305. Elbow pain & tennis elbow = take arnica, apply arnica cream to the affected area to help reduce inflammation and pain. Dosage: apply arnica cream to the affected area 2-3 times daily.

306. Electrolyte imbalance & mineral deficiency = take coconut water, drink coconut water to help restore electrolyte balance. Dosage: drink 8-16 ounces of coconut water daily.

307. Emphysema & lung damage = take mullein, make a tea from dried mullein leaves or consume mullein supplements to support lung health. Dosage: drink 1 cup of mullein tea 2-3 times or take 300-600 mg of mullein supplements daily.

308. Encephalitis & brain inflammation = take turmeric, use turmeric powder in cooking or make a tea with turmeric and black pepper to help manage encephalitis. Dosage: drink 1 cup of turmeric tea 2-3 times daily or take 500-2,000 mg of turmeric supplements daily.

309. Endocarditis = use garlic for its antimicrobial properties. Dosage: consume 1-2 cloves of raw garlic daily or take 600-1,200 mg of garlic supplements daily.

310. Endocarditis & heart infection = take garlic, consume raw garlic or garlic supplements to help manage endocarditis. Dosage: eat 2-3 raw garlic cloves daily or take 600-1,200 mg of garlic supplements daily.

311. Endometriosis & pelvic pain = take turmeric, use turmeric powder in cooking or make a tea with turmeric and black

pepper for anti-inflammatory effects to help manage endometriosis. Dosage: drink 1 cup of turmeric tea 2-3 times daily or take 500-2,000 mg of turmeric supplements daily.

312. Endometriosis & uterine tissue growth = take ginger, make a tea from fresh ginger to help manage endometriosis symptoms. Dosage: drink 1 cup of ginger tea 2-3 times daily.

313. Energy and cognitive function = take ginseng, brew roots in hot water for a tea or take in supplement form to boost energy and cognitive function. Dosage: drink 1 cup of ginseng tea 1-2 times daily or take 100-200 mg of ginseng supplements daily.

314. Energy and hormonal balance = take maca root, add powdered root to smoothies or food for boosting energy and supporting hormonal balance. Dosage: take 1-3 teaspoons of maca root powder daily.

315. Enlarged spleen & splenomegaly = take dandelion, make a tea from dried dandelion leaves or consume dandelion supplements to support spleen health. Dosage: drink 1 cup of dandelion tea 2-3 times daily or take 500-1,000 mg of dandelion supplements daily.

316. Epidermolysis bullosa = take calendula for wound healing. Dosage: apply calendula ointment or cream to affected areas 2-3 times daily.

317. Epididymitis & testicle inflammation = take saw palmetto, consume saw palmetto supplements to help manage epididymitis. Dosage: take 320 mg of saw palmetto supplements daily.

318. Epiglottitis & throat inflammation = take licorice root, make a tea from dried licorice root to help soothe the throat and manage epiglottitis. Dosage: drink 1 cup of licorice root tea 2-3 times daily.

319. Epilepsy = take lavender, use lavender essential oil in aromatherapy or make a tea from dried lavender flowers to help manage epilepsy symptoms. Dosage: drink 1 cup of lavender tea 1-2 times daily

or inhale lavender essential oil for 10-15 minutes daily.

320. Epstein-barr virus & viral infection = take elderberry, make a tea from dried elderberries or consume elderberry syrup to help manage epstein-barr virus. Dosage: drink 1 cup of elderberry tea 2-3 times daily or take 1 tablespoon of elderberry syrup 2-3 times daily.

321. Erectile dysfunction = take ginkgo biloba, make a tea from dried ginkgo biloba leaves or consume ginkgo biloba supplements to help manage erectile dysfunction. Dosage: drink 1 cup of ginkgo biloba tea 2-3 times daily or take 120-240 mg of ginkgo biloba supplements daily.

322. Erythema multiforme & skin condition = take calendula, apply calendula ointment to the affected area to help soothe erythema multiforme. Dosage: apply calendula ointment to the affected area 2-3 times daily.

323. Escherichia coli (e. Coli) infection & bacterial infection = take cranberry, consume cranberry juice or supplements to help manage e. Coli infections. Dosage: drink 8 ounces of cranberry juice daily or take 400-500 mg of cranberry supplements daily.

324. Esophagitis & esophageal inflammation = take slippery elm, make a tea from dried slippery elm bark or consume slippery elm supplements to help soothe esophageal inflammation. Dosage: drink 1 cup of slippery elm tea 2-3 times daily or take 400-800 mg of slippery elm supplements daily.

325. Essential tremor & shaking = take passionflower, consume passionflower supplements or make a tea from dried passionflower to help manage tremors. Dosage: drink 1 cup of passionflower tea 2-3 times daily or take 200-400 mg of passionflower supplements daily.

326. Eustachian tube dysfunction & ear health = take mullein, make a tea from dried mullein leaves and use as ear drops to help manage eustachian tube dysfunction. Dosage: drink 1 cup of mullein tea 2-3

times daily or use a few drops of mullein oil in the affected ear daily.

327. Excessive sweating & hyperhidrosis = take sage, make a tea from dried sage leaves to help reduce excessive sweating. Dosage: drink 1 cup of sage tea 2-3 times daily.

328. Exercise-induced asthma & respiratory condition = take ginger, make a tea from fresh ginger to help manage exercise-induced asthma. Dosage: drink 1 cup of ginger tea 2-3 times daily.

329. Eye floaters & vision condition = take bilberry, consume bilberry supplements or make a tea from dried bilberry leaves to help manage eye floaters. Dosage: drink 1 cup of bilberry tea 2-3 times daily or take 160-240 mg of bilberry supplements daily.

330. Eye strain & computer vision syndrome = take bilberry, consume bilberry supplements or make a tea from dried bilberry leaves to support eye health. Dosage: drink 1 cup of bilberry tea 2-3

times daily or take 160-240 mg of bilberry supplements daily.

331. Facial paralysis & bell's palsy = take st. John's wort, make a tea from dried st. John's wort flowers or consume st. John's wort supplements to help manage facial paralysis. Dosage: drink 1 cup of St. John's wort tea 2-3 times daily or take 300 mg of St. John's wort supplements 2-3 times daily.

332. Facial tics & spasms = take chamomile, make a tea from dried chamomile flowers or use chamomile essential oil in a bath to help relax muscles. Dosage: drink 1 cup of chamomile tea 2-3 times daily or add a few drops of chamomile essential oil to a warm bath.

333. Fainting & syncope = take hawthorn, make a tea from dried hawthorn berries or consume hawthorn supplements to help support heart health. Dosage: drink 1 cup of hawthorn tea 2-3 times daily or take 160-900 mg of hawthorn supplements daily.

334. Fatigue = take ginseng, consume ginseng root or make a tea to help manage fatigue. Dosage: drink 1 cup of ginseng tea 1-2 times daily or take 100-200 mg of ginseng supplements daily.

335. Fatigue & chronic exhaustion = take ashwagandha, consume ashwagandha supplements to help support energy levels. Dosage: take 300-500 mg of ashwagandha supplements daily.

336. Fatty liver disease & hepatic steatosis = take milk thistle, consume milk thistle supplements to support liver health and help manage fatty liver disease. Dosage: take 140-420 mg of milk thistle supplements daily.

337. Fecal incontinence & bowel control = take psyllium husk, consume psyllium husk supplements to help manage fecal incontinence. Dosage: take 5-10 grams of psyllium husk in water or juice daily.

338. Fever = take yarrow, steep dried leaves and flowers in hot water for 10 minutes to make a tea to reduce fever. Dosage: drink 1 cup of yarrow tea 2-3 times daily.

339. Fever blisters = take lemon balm, apply lemon balm cream or ointment to fever blisters to help manage symptoms. Dosage: apply lemon balm cream or ointment to the affected area 2-3 times daily.

340. Fibroadenoma & breast tissue growth = take turmeric, use turmeric powder in cooking or make a tea with turmeric and black pepper to help manage fibroadenoma. Dosage: drink 1 cup of turmeric tea 2-3 times daily or take 500-2,000 mg of turmeric supplements daily.

341. Fibrocystic breast disease & breast condition = take evening primrose oil, consume evening primrose oil supplements to help manage fibrocystic breast disease. Dosage: take 1,000-2,000 mg of evening primrose oil supplements daily.

342. Fibrocystic breast disease & breast lumps = take evening primrose oil, consume evening primrose oil supplements to help manage fibrocystic breast disease.

Dosage: take 1,000-2,000 mg of evening primrose oil supplements daily.

343. Fibromyalgia = take St. John's wort, make a tea from dried St. John's wort flowers or use St. John's wort oil topically to help manage fibromyalgia symptoms. Dosage: drink 1 cup of St. John's wort tea 2-3 times daily or apply St. John's wort oil to the affected area 2-3 times daily.

344. Fibromyalgia & chronic pain = take St. John's wort, make a tea from dried St. John's wort flowers or consume St. John's wort supplements to help manage fibromyalgia. Dosage: drink 1 cup of St. John's wort tea 2-3 times daily or take 300 mg of St. John's wort supplements 2-3 times daily.

345. Fistula & abnormal connection = take turmeric, apply turmeric paste to the affected area to help manage fistula. Dosage: apply turmeric paste to the affected area 2-3 times daily.

346. Flatulence = take caraway, chew caraway seeds or make a tea from the seeds to reduce gas and bloating. Dosage: chew 1 teaspoon of caraway seeds after meals or drink 1 cup of caraway tea 2-3 times daily.

347. Flatulence & excess gas = take fennel, chew fennel seeds or make a tea from dried fennel seeds to help relieve flatulence. Dosage: chew 1 teaspoon of fennel seeds after meals or drink 1 cup of fennel tea 2-3 times daily.

348. Flatulence & gas = take fennel seeds, chew on fennel seeds after meals to help manage flatulence. Dosage: chew 1 teaspoon of fennel seeds after meals or drink 1 cup of fennel tea 2-3 times daily.

349. Fleas & parasitic infestation = take neem oil, use neem oil spray or shampoo to help manage fleas. Dosage: apply neem oil spray or use neem oil shampoo on affected areas as needed.

350. Flu = take elderberry, consume elderberry syrup or make a tea from dried berries for flu symptoms. Dosage: drink 1 cup of elderberry tea 2-3 times daily or take 1 tablespoon of elderberry syrup 2-3 times daily.

351. Folic acid deficiency & nutritional deficiency = take spinach, consume spinach in salads or cooked dishes to help manage folic acid deficiency. Dosage: consume 1-2 cups of spinach daily.

352. Food poisoning & bacterial infections = take activated charcoal, consume activated charcoal supplements to help absorb toxins and manage food poisoning. Dosage: take 500-1,000 mg of activated charcoal supplements as needed, up to 4 times daily.

353. Food poisoning & digestive illness = take ginger, make a tea from fresh ginger to help manage symptoms of food poisoning. Dosage: drink 1 cup of ginger tea 2-3 times daily.

354. Foot fungus & athlete's foot = take tea tree oil, apply diluted tea tree oil to the affected areas to help manage foot fungus. Dosage: apply diluted tea tree oil to the affected area 2-3 times daily.

355. Fractures = take comfrey, apply comfrey ointment or poultice to fractured area to help promote healing. Dosage: apply comfrey ointment or poultice to the affected area 2-3 times daily.

356. Fractures & bone healing = take comfrey, apply comfrey cream or ointment to the affected areas to help promote bone healing. Dosage: apply comfrey cream or ointment to the affected area 2-3 times daily.

357. Fragile x syndrome & genetic disorder = take omega-3 fatty acids, consume fish oil supplements to help support brain health. Dosage: take 1,000-2,000 mg of fish oil supplements daily.

358. Frostbite = take cayenne pepper, apply cayenne pepper cream or ointment to affected areas to help manage frostbite. Dosage: apply cayenne pepper cream or ointment to the affected area 2-3 times daily.

359. Frozen shoulder = take turmeric, use turmeric powder in cooking or make a tea with turmeric and black pepper for anti-inflammatory effects to help manage frozen shoulder. Dosage: drink 1 cup of

turmeric tea 2-3 times daily or take 500-2,000 mg of turmeric supplements daily.

360. Frozen shoulder & adhesive capsulitis = take turmeric, use turmeric powder in cooking or make a tea with turmeric and black pepper to help manage inflammation. Dosage: drink 1 cup of turmeric tea 2-3 times daily or take 500-2,000 mg of turmeric supplements daily.

361. Frozen shoulder & shoulder stiffness = take turmeric, use turmeric powder in cooking or make a tea with turmeric and black pepper to help manage frozen shoulder. Dosage: drink 1 cup of turmeric tea 2-3 times daily or take 500-2,000 mg of turmeric supplements daily.

362. Fungal infections = take oregano oil, apply diluted oregano oil topically or consume internally to help manage fungal infections. Dosage: apply diluted oregano oil to the affected area 2-3 times daily or take 1-2 drops of oregano oil in a glass of water daily.

363. Fungal infections & ringworm = take garlic, apply crushed garlic directly to the affected areas or consume garlic supplements to help manage fungal infections. Dosage: apply crushed garlic to the affected area 2-3 times daily or take 600-1,200 mg of garlic supplements daily.

364. Fungal nail infection & onychomycosis = take tea tree oil, apply diluted tea tree oil to affected nails to help manage fungal infections. Dosage: apply diluted tea tree oil to the affected nails 2-3 times daily.

365. G6pd deficiency & enzyme deficiency = take ginkgo biloba, make a tea from dried ginkgo biloba leaves or consume ginkgo biloba supplements to help support enzyme function. Dosage: drink 1 cup of ginkgo biloba tea 1-2 times daily or take 120-240 mg of ginkgo biloba supplements daily.

366. Gallbladder cancer & biliary cancer = take dandelion, make a tea from dried dandelion leaves or consume dandelion supplements to help support gallbladder health. Dosage: drink 1 cup of dandelion tea 2-3 times daily or take 500 mg of dandelion root supplements daily.

367. Gallstones = take dandelion root, steep dried root in hot water for 10-15 minutes to make a tea to support liver health and aid in gallstone prevention. Dosage: drink 1 cup of dandelion root tea 2-3 times daily.

368. Gallstones & cholelithiasis = take dandelion, make a tea from dried dandelion leaves or consume dandelion supplements to support gallbladder health. Dosage: drink 1 cup of dandelion tea 2-3 times daily or take 500 mg of dandelion root supplements daily.

369. Ganglion cyst & joint lump = take frankincense oil, apply diluted frankincense oil to the affected area to help manage ganglion cysts. Dosage: apply diluted frankincense oil to the affected area 2-3 times daily.

370. Gangrene & tissue death = take echinacea, consume echinacea supplements or make a tea from dried echinacea to help boost the immune system. Dosage: drink 1 cup of echinacea tea 2-3 times daily or take 300-500 mg of echinacea supplements daily.

371. Gas & bloating = take peppermint, make a tea from dried peppermint leaves or chew fresh peppermint leaves to help relieve gas. Dosage: drink 1 cup of peppermint tea 2-3 times daily or chew fresh peppermint leaves as needed.

372. Gastric ulcer & stomach ulcer = take licorice root, make a tea from dried licorice root to help soothe gastric ulcers. Dosage: drink 1 cup of licorice root tea 2-3 times daily.

373. Gastritis = take chamomile, make a tea from dried chamomile flowers to help soothe gastritis symptoms. Dosage: drink 1 cup of chamomile tea 2-3 times daily.

374. Gastritis & stomach inflammation = take chamomile, make a tea from dried chamomile flowers to help soothe gastritis. Dosage: drink 1 cup of chamomile tea 2-3 times daily.

375. Gastroenteritis & stomach flu = take ginger, make a tea from fresh ginger to help manage gastroenteritis symptoms.

Dosage: drink 1 cup of ginger tea 2-3 times daily.

376. Gastroesophageal reflux disease (gerd) & acid reflux = take licorice root, make a tea from dried licorice root or consume licorice root supplements to help manage gerd. Dosage: drink 1 cup of licorice root tea 2-3 times daily or take 380-400 mg of deglycyrrhizinated licorice (dgl) supplements before meals.

377. Generalized anxiety disorder (gad) & anxiety = take kava kava, make a tea from dried kava kava root or consume kava kava supplements to help manage anxiety. Dosage: drink 1 cup of kava kava tea 1-2 times daily or take 100-250 mg of kava kava supplements daily.

378. Genital herpes & hsv infection = take lemon balm, apply lemon balm cream to the affected area to help manage genital herpes outbreaks. Dosage: apply lemon balm cream to the affected area 2-3 times daily.

379. Genital warts = take tea tree oil, apply diluted tea tree oil directly to affected areas to help manage genital warts. Dosage: apply diluted tea tree oil to the affected area 2-3 times daily.

380. Giant cell arteritis = use bromelain to reduce inflammation. Dosage: take 200-400 mg of bromelain supplements 2-3 times daily.

381. Gingivitis = take myrrh, rinse mouth with a myrrh-infused mouthwash to help reduce inflammation and treat gingivitis. Dosage: rinse mouth with myrrh-infused mouthwash 2-3 times daily.

382. Gingivitis & gum disease = take myrrh, use myrrh mouthwash or apply myrrh oil topically to help manage gum disease. Dosage: rinse mouth with myrrh-infused mouthwash 2-3 times daily or apply myrrh oil to the gums 2-3 times daily.

383. Gingivitis & gum inflammation = take myrrh, make a mouth rinse with myrrh tincture or powder to help manage gingivitis. Dosage: rinse mouth with myrrh-infused mouthwash 2-3 times daily.

384. Glaucoma = take bilberry, consume bilberry supplements or make a tea from dried bilberry leaves to help manage glaucoma symptoms. Dosage: drink 1 cup of bilberry tea 2-3 times daily or take 160 mg of bilberry supplements daily.

385. Glaucoma & eye pressure = take bilberry, make a tea from dried bilberry leaves or consume bilberry supplements to help manage glaucoma. Dosage: drink 1 cup of bilberry tea 2-3 times daily or take 160 mg of bilberry supplements daily.

386. Glaucoma & intraocular pressure = take bilberry, consume bilberry supplements or make a tea from dried bilberry leaves to support eye health. Dosage: drink 1 cup of bilberry tea 2-3 times daily or take 160 mg of bilberry supplements daily.

387. Glioblastoma & brain tumor = take turmeric, use turmeric powder in cooking or make a tea with turmeric and black pepper to help manage glioblastoma. Dosage: drink 1 cup of turmeric tea 2-3 times daily or take 500-2,000 mg of turmeric supplements daily.

388. Glomerulonephritis = consume nettle leaf to support kidney function. Dosage: drink 1-2 cups of nettle leaf tea daily or take 300-500 mg of nettle leaf supplements 2-3 times daily.

389. Glomerulonephritis & kidney inflammation = take parsley, make a tea from fresh parsley leaves or consume parsley supplements to help support kidney health. Dosage: drink 1 cup of parsley tea 2-3 times daily.

390. Goiter & enlarged thyroid = take bladderwrack, consume bladderwrack supplements to help manage thyroid health. Dosage: take 500 mg of bladderwrack supplements 1-2 times daily.

391. Gonorrhea & sexually transmitted infection = take goldenseal, make a tea from dried goldenseal root to help manage gonorrhea. Dosage: drink 1 cup of goldenseal tea 2-3 times daily.

392. Gout = take cherry extract, consume cherry juice or extract to help reduce gout flare-ups. Dosage: drink 1 cup of cherry

juice or take 1,000 mg of cherry extract daily.

393. Gout & joint inflammation = take tart cherry juice, drink tart cherry juice or consume tart cherry supplements to help manage gout. Dosage: drink 1 cup of tart cherry juice 2-3 times daily or take 1,000 mg of tart cherry supplements daily.

394. Gout & uric acid crystals = take cherry, consume fresh cherries or cherry juice to help manage gout. Dosage: drink 1 cup of cherry juice 2-3 times daily or eat 1-2 cups of fresh cherries daily.

395. Granuloma annulare & skin condition = take calendula, apply calendula ointment to the affected area to help soothe granuloma annulare. Dosage: apply calendula ointment to the affected area 2-3 times daily.

396. Granulomatosis with polyangiitis = take ginger to reduce inflammation and support immune function. Dosage: drink 1 cup of ginger tea 2-3 times daily or take 250-500 mg of ginger supplements 2-3 times daily.

397. Graves' disease & hyperthyroidism = take bugleweed, make a tea from dried bugleweed leaves or consume bugleweed supplements to help manage hyperthyroidism. Dosage: drink 1 cup of bugleweed tea 2-3 times daily or take 300-500 mg of bugleweed supplements daily.

398. Guillain-Barré syndrome = use St. John's wort to support nerve health. Dosage: take 300-600 mg of St. John's wort extract 2-3 times daily.

399. Guillain-barre syndrome & nerve damage = take st. John's wort, make a tea from dried st. John's wort flowers or consume st. John's wort supplements to help support nerve health. Dosage: drink 1 cup of st. John's wort tea 2-3 times daily or take 300-900 mg of st. John's wort supplements daily.

400. Guillain-barré syndrome & autoimmune disorder = take turmeric, use turmeric powder in cooking or make a tea with turmeric and black pepper to help manage guillain-barré syndrome. Dosage: drink 1 cup of turmeric tea 2-3 times daily or take

500-2,000 mg of turmeric supplements daily.

401. Gum disease & periodontitis = take tea tree oil, use tea tree oil mouthwash or toothpaste to help manage gum disease. Dosage: rinse mouth with tea tree oil mouthwash 2-3 times daily.

402. Gum disease (gingivitis) = take myrrh, rinse mouth with myrrh-infused mouthwash or apply myrrh oil to help manage gum disease. Dosage: rinse mouth with myrrh-infused mouthwash 2-3 times daily or apply myrrh oil to the gums 2-3 times daily.

403. Gum recession & periodontitis = take sage, make a tea from dried sage leaves or use sage mouthwash to help manage gum recession. Dosage: drink 1 cup of sage tea 2-3 times daily or rinse mouth with sage-infused mouthwash 2-3 times daily.

404. Hair loss = take saw palmetto, consume saw palmetto supplements or apply saw palmetto extract to the scalp to promote hair growth. Dosage: take 160-320 mg of saw palmetto supplements daily or apply saw palmetto extract to the scalp 1-2 times daily.

405. Hallucinations & psychotic disorder = take ginkgo biloba, make a tea from dried ginkgo biloba leaves or consume ginkgo biloba supplements to help support cognitive function. Dosage: drink 1 cup of ginkgo biloba tea 2-3 times daily or take 120-240 mg of ginkgo biloba supplements daily.

406. Hamstring injury & leg muscle strain = take arnica, apply arnica cream to the affected area to help reduce inflammation and pain. Dosage: apply arnica cream to the affected area 2-3 times daily.

407. Hand tremors & essential tremor = take valerian root, consume valerian root supplements or make a tea from dried valerian root to help manage hand tremors. Dosage: drink 1 cup of valerian root tea before bed or take 400-900 mg of valerian root supplements daily.

408. Hangnails = take calendula, apply calendula cream or ointment to affected areas to help manage hangnails. Dosage:

apply calendula cream to the affected area 2-3 times daily.

409. Hangover = take prickly pear cactus extract, consume prickly pear extract or juice to alleviate hangover symptoms. Dosage: take 1600 iu of prickly pear extract or drink 1 cup of prickly pear juice before consuming alcohol.

410. Hangover & alcohol detox = take ginger, make a tea from fresh ginger to help manage hangover symptoms. Dosage: drink 1 cup of ginger tea 2-3 times daily.

411. Hay fever = take butterbur, consume butterbur supplements or make a tea from dried butterbur root to help manage hay fever symptoms. Dosage: take 50-75 mg of butterbur supplements twice daily or drink 1 cup of butterbur tea 2 times daily.

412. Head lice = take tea tree oil, apply diluted tea tree oil to the scalp and hair to help manage head lice infestation. Dosage: apply diluted tea tree oil to the scalp and hair and leave it on for 30-40 minutes before rinsing; repeat daily until the infestation is cleared.

413. Headaches = take feverfew, consume fresh leaves or make a tea with dried feverfew leaves to help manage headaches. Dosage: drink 1 cup of feverfew tea 1-2 times daily or chew 1-2 fresh feverfew leaves daily.

414. Headaches and digestive issues = take peppermint, brew leaves in hot water for 10 minutes to make a tea for headaches or digestive issues. Dosage: drink 1 cup of peppermint tea 2-3 times daily.

415. Hearing loss = take ginkgo biloba, make a tea from dried ginkgo biloba leaves or consume ginkgo biloba supplements to help manage hearing loss. Dosage: drink 1 cup of ginkgo biloba tea 2-3 times daily or take 120-240 mg of ginkgo biloba supplements daily.

416. Hearing loss & tinnitus = take ginkgo biloba, make a tea from dried ginkgo biloba leaves or consume ginkgo biloba supplements to help manage tinnitus. Dosage: drink 1 cup of ginkgo biloba tea 2-3 times daily or take 120-240 mg of ginkgo biloba supplements daily.

417. Heart failure & cardiac condition = take garlic, consume raw garlic or garlic supplements to help support heart health. Dosage: take 600-1,200 mg of garlic supplements daily or use 1-2 cloves of fresh garlic daily.

418. Heart health = take hawthorn, brew berries in hot water for 10-15 minutes to make a tea for supporting heart health. Dosage: drink 1 cup of hawthorn tea 2-3 times daily.

419. Heart health and infections = take garlic, crush or chop fresh cloves and add to food, or take in supplement form for heart health and fighting infections. Dosage: take 600-1,200 mg of garlic supplements daily or use 1-2 cloves of fresh garlic daily.

420. Heart murmur & heart abnormality = take hawthorn, make a tea from dried hawthorn berries or consume hawthorn supplements to help support heart health. Dosage: drink 1 cup of hawthorn tea 2-3 times daily or take 160-900 mg of hawthorn supplements daily.

421. Heart palpitations & arrhythmia = take hawthorn, make a tea from dried hawthorn berries or consume hawthorn supplements to help manage heart palpitations. Dosage: drink 1 cup of hawthorn tea 2-3 times daily or take 160-900 mg of hawthorn supplements daily.

422. Heartburn = take slippery elm, make a tea from dried slippery elm bark or consume slippery elm supplements to help manage heartburn. Dosage: drink 1 cup of slippery elm tea 2-3 times daily or take 400-500 mg of slippery elm supplements before meals.

423. Heat stroke & heat exhaustion = take peppermint, make a tea from dried peppermint leaves to help cool the body and manage heat stroke. Dosage: drink 1 cup of peppermint tea 2-3 times daily.

424. Hemangioma & blood vessel tumor = take turmeric, use turmeric powder in cooking or make a tea with turmeric and black pepper to help manage hemangioma. Dosage: drink 1 cup of turmeric tea 2-3 times daily or use 1-2

teaspoons of turmeric powder in cooking daily.

425. Hematospermia & blood in semen = take saw palmetto, consume saw palmetto supplements to help manage hematospermia. Dosage: take 160-320 mg of saw palmetto supplements daily.

426. Hematuria & blood in urine = take cranberry, consume cranberry juice or supplements to help manage hematuria. Dosage: drink 1 cup of cranberry juice daily or take 500-1,500 mg of cranberry supplements daily.

427. Hemochromatosis = consume green tea to reduce iron absorption. Dosage: drink 2-3 cups of green tea daily.

428. Hemochromatosis & iron overload = take milk thistle, make a tea from dried milk thistle or consume milk thistle supplements to help support liver health. Dosage: drink 1 cup of milk thistle tea 2-3 times daily or take 150-450 mg of milk thistle supplements daily.

429. Hemolytic uremic syndrome = use cranberry to prevent urinary tract infections. Dosage: drink 1-2 cups of cranberry juice daily or take 500-1,000 mg of cranberry extract daily.

430. Hemophilia = use alfalfa to support blood clotting. Dosage: take 500-1,000 mg of alfalfa supplements daily or add fresh alfalfa sprouts to your diet.

431. Hemorrhage = take cayenne pepper, consume cayenne pepper in food or make a tea from dried cayenne pepper to help stop bleeding. Dosage: take 1/2 to 1 teaspoon of cayenne pepper in water or food as needed.

432. Hemorrhoids = take witch hazel, apply witch hazel cream or ointment to hemorrhoids for relief from itching and swelling. Dosage: apply witch hazel cream to the affected area 2-3 times daily.

433. Hemorrhoids & anal swelling = take witch hazel, apply witch hazel cream or pads to the affected area to help manage hemorrhoids. Dosage: apply witch hazel cream or pads to the affected area 2-3 times daily.

434. Hepatitis & liver inflammation = take milk thistle, consume milk thistle supplements to support liver health and help manage hepatitis. Dosage: take 200-400 mg of milk thistle supplements 2-3 times daily.

435. Hepatitis C = take licorice root for liver support. Dosage: drink 1-2 cups of licorice root tea daily or take 380-800 mg of licorice root extract daily.

436. Hereditary angioedema = use bromelain to reduce swelling. Dosage: take 500-1,000 mg of bromelain supplements 2-3 times daily.

437. Hernia & abdominal protrusion = take comfrey, apply comfrey cream or ointment to the affected areas to help manage hernia symptoms. Dosage: apply comfrey cream to the affected area 2-3 times daily.

438. Herpes simplex virus (hsv) = take lemon balm, apply lemon balm cream or ointment to herpes lesions to help manage symptoms. Dosage: apply lemon balm cream to the affected area 2-3 times daily.

439. Herpes zoster & shingles = take lemon balm, apply lemon balm ointment to the affected areas or make a tea from dried lemon balm leaves to help manage shingles. Dosage: apply lemon balm ointment to the affected area 2-3 times daily or drink 1 cup of lemon balm tea 2-3 times daily.

440. Hiccups & diaphragm spasms = take dill, make a tea from dried dill seeds to help manage hiccups. Dosage: drink 1 cup of dill tea as needed.

441. High blood pressure = take hibiscus, steep dried flowers in hot water for 10 minutes to make a tea to lower blood pressure. Dosage: drink 1 cup of hibiscus tea 2-3 times daily.

442. High cholesterol = take artichoke, consume artichoke extract or make a tea from dried leaves to help lower cholesterol levels. Dosage: drink 1 cup of artichoke tea 2-3 times daily or take 320-

640 mg of artichoke supplements 2-3 times daily.

443. High cholesterol & hyperlipidemia = take fenugreek, consume fenugreek supplements or make a tea from dried fenugreek seeds to help manage high cholesterol. Dosage: drink 1 cup of fenugreek tea 2-3 times daily or take 2-5 grams of fenugreek seeds or supplements daily.

444. Hirsutism & excess hair growth = take spearmint tea, drink spearmint tea regularly to help manage hirsutism. Dosage: drink 1 cup of spearmint tea 2 times daily.

445. Hives = take nettle, make a tea from dried nettle leaves or apply nettle cream to help manage hives. Dosage: drink 1 cup of nettle tea 2-3 times daily or apply nettle cream to the affected area as needed.

446. Hodgkin's lymphoma & lymphatic cancer = take turmeric, use turmeric powder in cooking or make a tea with turmeric and black pepper to help manage hodgkin's lymphoma. Dosage: drink 1 cup of turmeric tea 2-3 times daily or use 1-2 teaspoons of turmeric powder in cooking daily.

447. Hot flashes = take black cohosh, consume black cohosh supplements or make a tea from dried roots to alleviate hot flashes. Dosage: take 20-40 mg of black cohosh supplements 1-2 times daily.

448. Hot flashes & menopausal symptoms = take black cohosh, consume black cohosh supplements to help manage hot flashes. Dosage: take 20-40 mg of black cohosh supplements 1-2 times daily.

449. Hydrocephalus & brain condition = take gotu kola, consume gotu kola supplements to help support brain health. Dosage: take 500-1,000 mg of gotu kola supplements daily.

450. Hyperacidity & stomach ulcers = take licorice root, make a tea from dried licorice root or consume licorice root supplements to help manage hyperacidity. Dosage: drink 1 cup of licorice root tea 2-3 times daily or take 380-400 mg of

deglycyrrhizinated licorice (dgl) supplements before meals.

451. Hyperactivity = take passionflower, make a tea from dried passionflower leaves and flowers to calm hyperactivity. Dosage: drink 1 cup of passionflower tea 2-3 times daily.

452. Hyperaldosteronism = take dandelion to support kidney function and reduce blood pressure. Dosage: drink 1 cup of dandelion tea 2-3 times daily or take 500-1,000 mg of dandelion root extract daily.

453. Hyperglycemia & high blood sugar = take cinnamon, use cinnamon powder in cooking or consume cinnamon supplements to help manage high blood sugar. Dosage: take 1-6 grams of cinnamon powder or supplements daily.

454. Hyperhidrosis & excessive sweating = take sage, make a tea from dried sage leaves to help reduce excessive sweating. Dosage: drink 1 cup of sage tea 2-3 times daily.

455. Hyperkalemia & high potassium levels = take dandelion, make a tea from dried dandelion leaves or consume dandelion supplements to help manage potassium levels. Dosage: drink 1 cup of dandelion tea 2-3 times daily or take 500 mg of dandelion root supplements daily.

456. Hyperlipidemia & high blood fat levels = take artichoke, consume artichoke supplements or make a tea from dried artichoke leaves to help manage high blood fat levels. Dosage: drink 1 cup of artichoke tea 2-3 times daily or take 320-640 mg of artichoke supplements 2-3 times daily.

457. Hypersensitivity pneumonitis = use butterbur to reduce lung inflammation. Dosage: take 50-100 mg of butterbur extract 2-3 times daily.

458. Hypertension = take garlic, consume garlic supplements or use garlic in cooking to help lower blood pressure. Dosage: take 600-1,200 mg of garlic supplements daily or use 1-2 cloves of fresh garlic daily.

459. Hypertension & high blood pressure = take hibiscus, make a tea from dried

hibiscus flowers to help manage high blood pressure. Dosage: drink 1 cup of hibiscus tea 2-3 times daily.

460. Hyperthyroidism = take bugleweed, make a tea from dried bugleweed leaves to help manage symptoms of hyperthyroidism. Dosage: drink 1 cup of bugleweed tea 2-3 times daily.

461. Hyperthyroidism & overactive thyroid = take lemon balm, make a tea from dried lemon balm leaves to help manage hyperthyroidism. Dosage: drink 1 cup of lemon balm tea 2-3 times daily.

462. Hypocalcemia & low calcium levels = take alfalfa, consume alfalfa supplements or make a tea from dried alfalfa leaves to help increase calcium levels. Dosage: drink 1 cup of alfalfa tea 2-3 times daily or take 500-1,000 mg of alfalfa supplements daily.

463. Hypoglycemia = take cinnamon, sprinkle cinnamon on food or make a tea from cinnamon powder to help manage hypoglycemia. Dosage: take 1-6 grams of cinnamon powder daily.

464. Hypoglycemia & low blood sugar = take licorice root, make a tea from dried licorice root or consume licorice root supplements to help manage low blood sugar. Dosage: drink 1 cup of licorice root tea 2-3 times daily or take 380-400 mg of deglycyrrhizinated licorice (dgl) supplements before meals.

465. Hypokalemia & low potassium levels = take dandelion, make a tea from dried dandelion leaves or consume dandelion supplements to help manage potassium levels. Dosage: drink 1 cup of dandelion tea 2-3 times daily or take 500 mg of dandelion root supplements daily.

466. Hyponatremia & low sodium levels = take dandelion, make a tea from dried dandelion leaves or consume dandelion supplements to help manage sodium levels. Dosage: drink 1 cup of dandelion tea 2-3 times daily or take 500 mg of dandelion root supplements daily.

467. Hypoparathyroidism = use nettle to help balance calcium levels. Dosage: drink 1

cup of nettle tea 2-3 times daily or take 300-600 mg of nettle supplements daily.

468. Hypospadias = take aloe vera, apply fresh aloe vera gel to help manage hypospadias. Dosage: apply fresh aloe vera gel to the affected area 2-3 times daily.

469. Hypotension (low blood pressure) = take licorice root, chew on licorice root or make a tea from dried licorice root to help manage hypotension. Dosage: drink 1 cup of licorice root tea 2-3 times daily or chew on a small piece of licorice root as needed.

470. Hypothyroidism = take ashwagandha, consume ashwagandha supplements or make a tea from dried ashwagandha root to help support thyroid function in hypothyroidism. Dosage: drink 1 cup of ashwagandha tea 2-3 times daily or take 300-500 mg of ashwagandha supplements daily.

471. Hypothyroidism & underactive thyroid = take ashwagandha, consume ashwagandha supplements to help support thyroid function. Dosage: take

300-600 mg of ashwagandha supplements daily.

472. Ibuprofen overdose & nsaid toxicity = take milk thistle, make a tea from dried milk thistle or consume milk thistle supplements to help support liver health. Dosage: drink 1 cup of milk thistle tea 2-3 times daily or take 150-450 mg of milk thistle supplements daily.

473. Idiopathic pulmonary fibrosis = consume cordyceps to improve lung function. Dosage: take 1,000-3,000 mg of cordyceps extract daily.

474. Immune system and energy levels = take astragalus, simmer roots in water for 30 minutes to make a tea for strengthening the immune system and supporting energy levels. Dosage: drink 1 cup of astragalus tea 2-3 times daily or take 250-500 mg of astragalus supplements daily.

475. Immune system and stress = take reishi mushroom, simmer dried mushrooms in water for 30 minutes to make a tea for boosting the immune system and

reducing stress. Dosage: drink 1 cup of reishi mushroom tea 1-2 times daily.

476. Immune system support = take echinacea, consume echinacea supplements or make a tea from dried echinacea roots to support immune function. Dosage: take 300-500 mg of echinacea supplements 2-3 times daily or drink 1 cup of echinacea tea 2-3 times daily.

477. Impetigo = take goldenseal, apply goldenseal cream or ointment to affected areas to help manage impetigo. Dosage: apply goldenseal cream to the affected area 2-3 times daily.

478. Impetigo & bacterial skin infection = take tea tree oil, apply diluted tea tree oil to the affected skin area to help manage impetigo. Dosage: apply diluted tea tree oil to the affected area 2-3 times daily.

479. Impetigo & skin infection = take tea tree oil, apply diluted tea tree oil to the affected areas to help manage impetigo. Dosage: apply diluted tea tree oil to the affected areas 2-3 times daily.

480. Impotence = take ginkgo biloba, make a tea from dried leaves or consume ginkgo biloba supplements to improve blood flow. Dosage: drink 1 cup of ginkgo biloba tea 2-3 times daily or take 120-240 mg of ginkgo biloba supplements daily.

481. Impotence (erectile dysfunction) = take ginseng, consume ginseng root or make a tea to help manage impotence. Dosage: take 200-400 mg of ginseng supplements daily or drink 1 cup of ginseng tea 2 times daily.

482. Incontinence & bladder control = take corn silk, make a tea from dried corn silk to help support bladder health and manage incontinence. Dosage: drink 1 cup of corn silk tea 2-3 times daily.

483. Indigestion = take ginger, chew raw ginger or make a tea from fresh ginger slices to help manage indigestion. Dosage: drink 1 cup of ginger tea 2-3 times daily or chew a small piece of raw ginger before meals.

484. Indigestion & dyspepsia = take peppermint, make a tea from dried

peppermint leaves or chew fresh peppermint leaves to help manage indigestion. Dosage: drink 1 cup of peppermint tea 2-3 times daily or chew fresh peppermint leaves after meals.

485. Infantile colic & baby's intestinal pain = take fennel, make a tea from fennel seeds to help manage infantile colic. Dosage: drink 1 cup of fennel tea 2-3 times daily.

486. Infertility = take maca root, consume maca root powder or supplements to help support fertility and reproductive health. Dosage: take 1,500-3,000 mg of maca root supplements daily or use 1-2 teaspoons of maca root powder daily.

487. Infertility & conception issues = take maca root, consume maca root supplements to help support fertility. Dosage: take 1,500-3,000 mg of maca root supplements daily.

488. Inflammation = take boswellia, consume boswellia supplements or use boswellia extract to reduce inflammation. Dosage: take 300-500 mg of boswellia supplements 2-3 times daily.

489. Inflammatory bowel disease (ibd) & chronic bowel inflammation = take turmeric, use turmeric powder in cooking or make a tea with turmeric and black pepper to help manage inflammation in ibd. Dosage: drink 1 cup of turmeric tea 2-3 times daily or use 1-2 teaspoons of turmeric powder in cooking daily.

490. Influenza = take elderberry, consume elderberry syrup or make a tea from dried elderberries to help manage influenza symptoms. Dosage: take 1 tablespoon of elderberry syrup 2-3 times daily or drink 1 cup of elderberry tea 2-3 times daily.

491. Ingrown hair = take tea tree oil, apply diluted tea tree oil directly to affected areas to help manage ingrown hairs. Dosage: apply diluted tea tree oil to affected areas 2-3 times daily.

492. Ingrown toenail = take tea tree oil, apply diluted tea tree oil directly to the affected toenail to help manage ingrown toenails. Dosage: apply diluted tea tree oil to the affected toenail 2-3 times daily.

493. Ingrown toenails & nail infections = take tea tree oil, apply diluted tea tree oil to the affected areas to help manage ingrown toenails. Dosage: apply diluted tea tree oil to the affected areas 2-3 times daily.

494. Insect bites = take calendula, apply calendula cream or ointment to insect bites to help soothe irritation. Dosage: apply calendula cream to insect bites 2-3 times daily.

495. Insomnia = take valerian root, steep dried root in hot water for 10-15 minutes to make a tea for better sleep. Dosage: drink 1 cup of valerian root tea before bed or take 400-900 mg of valerian root supplements daily.

496. Insomnia & sleep disorders = take valerian root, consume valerian root supplements or make a tea from dried valerian root to help manage insomnia. Dosage: drink 1 cup of valerian root tea before bed or take 400-900 mg of valerian root supplements daily.

497. Interstitial cystitis = take marshmallow root, steep dried marshmallow root in hot water for 10 minutes to make a soothing tea for interstitial cystitis. Dosage: drink 1 cup of marshmallow root tea 2-3 times daily.

498. Interstitial cystitis & bladder pain = take marshmallow root, make a tea from dried marshmallow root to help soothe the bladder. Dosage: drink 1 cup of marshmallow root tea 2-3 times daily.

499. Intestinal worms & parasites = take wormwood, make a tea from dried wormwood leaves or consume wormwood supplements to help manage intestinal worms. Dosage: drink 1 cup of wormwood tea 1-2 times daily or take 200-400 mg of wormwood supplements daily.

500. Irritable bowel syndrome (ibs) = take peppermint oil, consume enteric-coated peppermint oil capsules to alleviate symptoms of ibs. Dosage: take 1-2 enteric-coated peppermint oil capsules 2-3 times daily.

501. Irritable bowel syndrome (ibs) & digestive issues = take peppermint, make a tea from

dried peppermint leaves or chew fresh peppermint leaves to help manage ibs. Dosage: drink 1 cup of peppermint tea 2-3 times daily or chew fresh peppermint leaves after meals.

502. Ischemic stroke & brain blood flow = take ginkgo biloba, make a tea from dried ginkgo biloba leaves or consume ginkgo biloba supplements to help support brain blood flow. Dosage: drink 1 cup of ginkgo biloba tea 1-2 times daily or take 120-240 mg of ginkgo biloba supplements daily.

503. Itching = take chamomile, apply chamomile cream or make a tea from dried chamomile flowers to relieve itching. Dosage: apply chamomile cream to the affected area 2-3 times daily or drink 1 cup of chamomile tea 2-3 times daily.

504. Jaundice = take dandelion root, steep dried dandelion root in hot water for 10-15 minutes to make a tea to support liver function and help manage jaundice. Dosage: drink 1 cup of dandelion root tea 2-3 times daily.

505. Jaundice & liver condition = take dandelion root, make a tea from dried dandelion root to help support liver function. Dosage: drink 1 cup of dandelion root tea 2-3 times daily.

506. Joint pain = take ginger, use ginger in cooking or make a tea from fresh ginger to reduce joint pain and inflammation. Dosage: drink 1 cup of ginger tea 2-3 times daily or use 1-2 teaspoons of fresh ginger in cooking daily.

507. Kawasaki disease & childhood vasculitis = take ginger, make a tea from fresh ginger to help manage inflammation in kawasaki disease. Dosage: drink 1 cup of ginger tea 2-3 times daily.

508. Keloids = take aloe vera, apply fresh aloe vera gel directly to keloids to help reduce inflammation and promote healing. Dosage: apply fresh aloe vera gel to keloids 2-3 times daily.

509. Keratitis & corneal inflammation = take chamomile, make a tea from dried chamomile flowers and use as an eye wash to help manage keratitis. Dosage: use

chamomile tea as an eye wash 2-3 times daily.

510. Kidney cancer & renal tumor = take milk thistle, make a tea from dried milk thistle or consume milk thistle supplements to help support kidney health. Dosage: drink 1 cup of milk thistle tea 2-3 times daily or take 150-450 mg of milk thistle supplements daily.

511. Kidney stones = take hydrangea root, steep dried root in hot water for 10-15 minutes to make a tea to support kidney health and aid in kidney stone prevention. Dosage: drink 1 cup of hydrangea root tea 2-3 times daily.

512. Kidney stones & nephrolithiasis = take chanca piedra, make a tea from dried chanca piedra leaves to help manage kidney stones. Dosage: drink 1 cup of chanca piedra tea 2-3 times daily.

513. Kidney stones & renal calculi = take hydrangea root, make a tea from dried hydrangea root to help manage kidney stones. Dosage: drink 1 cup of hydrangea root tea 2-3 times daily.

514. Klinefelter syndrome & chromosomal disorder = take maca root, consume maca root supplements to help support hormone balance. Dosage: take 1,500-3,000 mg of maca root supplements daily.

515. Labyrinthitis & inner ear inflammation = take ginger, make a tea from fresh ginger to help manage inflammation in labyrinthitis. Dosage: drink 1 cup of ginger tea 2-3 times daily.

516. Lactation issues & low milk supply = take fenugreek, consume fenugreek supplements or make a tea from dried fenugreek seeds to help increase milk supply. Dosage: take 1,500-3,000 mg of fenugreek supplements daily or drink 1 cup of fenugreek tea 2-3 times daily.

517. Lactose intolerance = take lactase enzyme supplements, consume lactase enzyme before consuming dairy products to aid digestion. Dosage: follow the dosage instructions on the lactase enzyme supplement packaging before consuming dairy.

518. Laryngitis & voice box inflammation = take licorice root, make a tea from dried licorice root to help soothe the throat and manage laryngitis. Dosage: drink 1 cup of licorice root tea 2-3 times daily.

519. Laryngitis & voice loss = take licorice root, make a tea from dried licorice root to help soothe the throat and manage laryngitis. Dosage: drink 1 cup of licorice root tea 2-3 times daily.

520. Lead poisoning & heavy metal toxicity = take cilantro, consume cilantro in salads or dishes to help support detoxification from lead poisoning. Dosage: include 1-2 tablespoons of fresh cilantro in your daily diet.

521. Leaky gut syndrome & intestinal permeability = take slippery elm, make a tea from dried slippery elm bark or consume slippery elm supplements to help soothe the digestive tract. Dosage: drink 1 cup of slippery elm tea 2-3 times daily or take 400-600 mg of slippery elm supplements daily.

522. Leg cramps = take magnesium, consume magnesium-rich foods or supplements to help manage leg cramps. Dosage: consume 300-400 mg of magnesium supplements daily or include magnesium-rich foods like nuts, seeds, and leafy greens in your diet.

523. Leg cramps & muscle spasms = take magnesium, consume magnesium-rich foods or supplements to help manage leg cramps. Dosage: consume 300-400 mg of magnesium supplements daily or include magnesium-rich foods like nuts, seeds, and leafy greens in your diet.

524. Leishmaniasis & parasitic infection = take neem, make a tea from dried neem leaves or consume neem supplements to help manage leishmaniasis. Dosage: drink 1 cup of neem tea 1-2 times daily or take 300-600 mg of neem supplements daily.

525. Leukemia = take turmeric, use turmeric powder in cooking or make a tea with turmeric and black pepper for anti-inflammatory effects to support leukemia management. Dosage: take 500-2,000 mg

of turmeric supplements daily or use 1-2 teaspoons of turmeric powder in cooking daily.

526. Leukemia & blood cancer = take green tea, drink green tea regularly to provide antioxidant support to help manage leukemia. Dosage: drink 2-3 cups of green tea daily.

527. Lice = take tea tree oil, apply diluted tea tree oil to the scalp and hair to help manage lice infestation. Dosage: apply diluted tea tree oil to the scalp and hair daily for a week, then repeat as necessary.

528. Lichen planus & skin rash = take aloe vera, apply aloe vera gel to the affected areas to help manage lichen planus. Dosage: apply aloe vera gel to the affected areas 2-3 times daily.

529. Liver cirrhosis = take milk thistle, consume milk thistle supplements or make a tea from dried milk thistle seeds to support liver health in cirrhosis. Dosage: take 150-450 mg of milk thistle supplements daily or drink 1 cup of milk thistle tea 2-3 times daily.

530. Liver cirrhosis & scarring = take milk thistle, consume milk thistle supplements to support liver health and help manage liver cirrhosis. Dosage: take 150-450 mg of milk thistle supplements daily.

531. Liver health and detoxification = take yellow dock, simmer roots in water for 15 minutes to make a tea for liver health and detoxification. Dosage: drink 1 cup of yellow dock tea 1-2 times daily.

532. Low back pain = take willow bark, steep dried willow bark in hot water for 10-15 minutes to make a tea to help manage low back pain. Dosage: drink 1 cup of willow bark tea 2-3 times daily.

533. Low libido = take horny goat weed, consume horny goat weed supplements or make a tea from dried leaves to support libido. Dosage: take 250-500 mg of horny goat weed supplements daily or drink 1 cup of horny goat weed tea daily.

534. Low libido & sexual dysfunction = take maca root, consume maca root supplements to help support libido.

Dosage: take 1,500-3,000 mg of maca root supplements daily.

535. Low sperm count & male infertility = take ashwagandha, consume ashwagandha supplements to help support sperm count. Dosage: take 300-500 mg of ashwagandha supplements twice daily.

536. Lumbago & lower back pain = take devil's claw, consume devil's claw supplements or make a tea from dried devil's claw root to help manage lower back pain. Dosage: take 600-1,200 mg of devil's claw supplements daily or drink 1 cup of devil's claw tea 1-2 times daily.

537. Lupus & autoimmune disease = take turmeric, use turmeric powder in cooking or make a tea with turmeric and black pepper to help manage lupus. Dosage: take 500-2,000 mg of turmeric supplements daily or use 1-2 teaspoons of turmeric powder in cooking daily.

538. Lyme disease & tick-borne illness = take cat's claw, consume cat's claw supplements to help manage lyme disease.

Dosage: take 250-1,000 mg of cat's claw supplements daily.

539. Lymphangioleiomyomatosis (LAM) = take red clover for its antioxidant properties. Dosage: drink 1-2 cups of red clover tea daily or take 40-160 mg of red clover extract 2-3 times daily.

540. Lymphedema = take dandelion root, steep dried dandelion root in hot water for 10-15 minutes to make a tea to help manage lymphedema. Dosage: drink 1 cup of dandelion root tea 2-3 times daily.

541. Macular degeneration & vision loss = take bilberry, consume bilberry supplements or make a tea from dried bilberry leaves to support eye health. Dosage: take 160-320 mg of bilberry supplements daily or drink 1 cup of bilberry tea 1-2 times daily.

542. Malaria & mosquito-borne illness = take artemisia annua (sweet wormwood), make a tea from dried artemisia annua leaves to help manage malaria. Dosage: drink 1 cup of artemisia annua tea 1-2 times daily.

543. Marfan syndrome = use gotu kola to support connective tissue health. Dosage:

take 500-1,000 mg of gotu kola extract 2-3 times daily.

544. Measles = take elderberry, consume elderberry syrup or make a tea from dried elderberries to help manage measles symptoms. Dosage: take 1-2 teaspoons of elderberry syrup 2-3 times daily or drink 1 cup of elderberry tea 2-3 times daily.

545. Melasma = take licorice root, apply licorice root cream or make a tea from dried licorice root to help manage melasma. Dosage: apply licorice root cream to affected areas twice daily or drink 1 cup of licorice root tea 1-2 times daily.

546. Melasma & skin pigmentation = take turmeric, apply a paste made from turmeric powder and water to the affected areas to help manage melasma. Dosage: apply turmeric paste to affected areas once daily and leave for 10-15 minutes before rinsing off.

547. Memory and concentration = take rosemary, steep fresh or dried leaves in hot water for 10 minutes to enhance memory and concentration. Dosage: drink 1 cup of rosemary tea 1-2 times daily.

548. Memory loss = take ginkgo biloba, make a tea from dried leaves to enhance memory and cognitive function. Dosage: drink 1 cup of ginkgo biloba tea 1-2 times daily or take 120-240 mg of ginkgo biloba supplements daily.

549. Meniere's disease & inner ear disorder = take ginger, chew raw ginger or make a tea from fresh ginger to help manage meniere's disease. Dosage: chew a small piece of raw ginger or drink 1 cup of ginger tea 1-2 times daily.

550. Menopause = take red clover, make a tea from dried red clover flowers to help alleviate menopausal symptoms. Dosage: drink 1 cup of red clover tea 1-2 times daily.

551. Menorrhagia & heavy menstrual bleeding = take shepherd's purse, make a tea from dried shepherd's purse leaves to help manage heavy menstrual bleeding.

Dosage: drink 1 cup of shepherd's purse tea 1-2 times daily.

552. Menstrual cramps = take cramp bark, steep dried bark in hot water for 10-15 minutes to make a tea for menstrual cramp relief. Dosage: drink 1 cup of cramp bark tea 1-2 times daily.

553. Menstrual irregularities = take dong quai, make a tea from dried dong quai root to help manage menstrual irregularities. Dosage: drink 1 cup of dong quai tea 1-2 times daily.

554. Metabolism and pain = take cayenne pepper, add a pinch to food or mix with warm water for a metabolism boost and pain relief. Dosage: add a pinch of cayenne pepper to food daily or mix 1/4 teaspoon in warm water once daily.

555. Migraine = take feverfew, consume fresh leaves or make a tea with dried leaves for migraine headache relief. Dosage: chew 1-2 fresh feverfew leaves daily or drink 1 cup of feverfew tea 1-2 times daily.

556. Miscarriage prevention & pregnancy support = take raspberry leaf, make a tea from dried raspberry leaves to help support pregnancy. Dosage: drink 1 cup of raspberry leaf tea 1-2 times daily.

557. Motion sickness = take ginger, chew raw ginger or make a tea from fresh ginger slices to help manage motion sickness. Dosage: chew a small piece of raw ginger or drink 1 cup of ginger tea 1-2 times daily.

558. Mouth sores = take chamomile, apply chamomile cream or make a tea from dried chamomile flowers to help manage mouth sores. Dosage: apply chamomile cream to affected areas 2-3 times daily or drink 1 cup of chamomile tea 2-3 times daily.

559. Mouth ulcers = take licorice root, chew on licorice root or make a tea from dried licorice root to help manage mouth ulcers. Dosage: chew a small piece of licorice root several times daily or drink 1 cup of licorice root tea 1-2 times daily.

560. Mouth ulcers & canker sores = use licorice root to reduce inflammation and promote healing. Dosage: drink 1 cup of

licorice root tea 2-3 times daily or take 300-600 mg of licorice root extract daily. You can also apply a paste made from licorice root powder and water directly to the sores 2-3 times daily.

561. Multiple sclerosis & neurodegenerative disease = take ginkgo biloba, make a tea from dried ginkgo biloba leaves or consume ginkgo biloba supplements to help support brain function and manage symptoms of multiple sclerosis. Dosage: drink 1 cup of ginkgo biloba tea 1-2 times daily or take 120-240 mg of ginkgo biloba supplements daily.

562. Multiple sclerosis (ms) & nerve damage = take ginkgo biloba, make a tea from dried ginkgo biloba leaves or consume ginkgo biloba supplements to help support nerve health. Dosage: drink 1 cup of ginkgo biloba tea 1-2 times daily or take 120-240 mg of ginkgo biloba supplements daily.

563. Muscle cramps = take magnesium, consume magnesium-rich foods or supplements to prevent muscle cramps. Dosage: take 300-400 mg of magnesium supplements daily or include magnesium-rich foods like nuts, seeds, and leafy greens in your diet.

564. Muscle soreness & post-exercise pain = take magnesium, consume magnesium-rich foods or supplements to help manage muscle soreness. Dosage: take 300-400 mg of magnesium supplements daily or include magnesium-rich foods like nuts, seeds, and leafy greens in your diet.

565. Muscular dystrophy & muscle weakness = take creatine, consume creatine supplements to help support muscle strength. Dosage: take 3-5 grams of creatine supplements daily.

566. Myasthenia gravis = consume ashwagandha to improve muscle strength. Dosage: take 300-600 mg of ashwagandha extract 2-3 times daily.

567. Myasthenia gravis & muscle weakness = take ginseng, consume ginseng supplements or make a tea from dried ginseng root to help manage muscle weakness. Dosage: take 200-400 mg of

ginseng supplements daily or drink 1 cup of ginseng tea 1-2 times daily.

568. Myasthenia gravis & neuromuscular disorder = take astragalus root, make a tea from dried astragalus root or consume astragalus supplements to help support immune function and manage myasthenia gravis. Dosage: drink 1 cup of astragalus tea 1-2 times daily or follow supplement dosage recommendations.

569. Myopia = take eyebright, make a tea from dried eyebright leaves to help manage myopia (nearsightedness). Dosage: drink 1 cup of eyebright tea 1-2 times daily.

570. Nail fungus = take tea tree oil, apply diluted tea tree oil directly to affected nails to treat nail fungus. Dosage: apply diluted tea tree oil to affected nails twice daily.

571. Nail fungus & onychomycosis = take tea tree oil, apply diluted tea tree oil to the affected nails to help manage nail fungus. Dosage: apply diluted tea tree oil to affected nails twice daily.

572. Narcolepsy & excessive sleepiness = take ginseng, consume ginseng supplements or make a tea from dried ginseng root to help manage narcolepsy. Dosage: take 200-400 mg of ginseng supplements daily or drink 1 cup of ginseng tea 1-2 times daily.

573. Nasal congestion = take eucalyptus, use eucalyptus oil in steam inhalation to help manage nasal congestion. Dosage: add a few drops of eucalyptus oil to hot water and inhale the steam for 5-10 minutes.

574. Nausea = take ginger, chew raw ginger or make a tea from fresh ginger slices to alleviate nausea. Dosage: chew a small piece of raw ginger or drink 1 cup of ginger tea as needed for nausea relief.

575. Necrotizing fasciitis = use echinacea to boost immune response. Dosage: take 300-600 mg of echinacea extract 2-3 times daily.

576. Nephritis & kidney inflammation = take nettle, make a tea from dried nettle leaves or consume nettle supplements to help manage nephritis. Dosage: drink 1 cup of nettle tea 1-2 times daily or follow supplement dosage recommendations.

577. Nephrotic syndrome & kidney disorder = take marshmallow root, make a tea from dried marshmallow root to help soothe and support kidney function in nephrotic syndrome. Dosage: drink 1 cup of marshmallow root tea 1-2 times daily.

578. Nerve pain = take st. John's wort, make a tea from dried flowers or use st. John's wort oil topically to alleviate nerve pain. Dosage: drink 1 cup of st. John's wort tea 1-2 times daily or apply st. John's wort oil to affected areas as needed.

579. Neuralgia = take st. John's wort, make a tea from dried st. John's wort flowers or use st. John's wort oil topically to help manage neuralgia. Dosage: drink 1 cup of st. John's wort tea 1-2 times daily or apply st. John's wort oil to affected areas as needed.

580. Neuralgia & nerve pain = take st. John's wort, make a tea from dried st. John's wort flowers or consume st. John's wort supplements to help manage nerve pain. Dosage: drink 1 cup of st. John's wort tea

1-2 times daily or take st. John's wort supplements as recommended.

581. Nightmares = take valerian root, steep dried valerian root in hot water for 10-15 minutes to make a tea to help manage nightmares. Dosage: drink 1 cup of valerian root tea 1 hour before bedtime.

582. Non-hodgkin's lymphoma & lymphatic cancer = take green tea, drink green tea regularly to provide antioxidant support to help manage non-hodgkin's lymphoma. Dosage: drink 2-3 cups of green tea daily.

583. Obesity = take green tea, steep dried green tea leaves in hot water for 3-5 minutes to aid in weight management. Dosage: drink 2-3 cups of green tea daily for weight management.

584. Obsessive-compulsive disorder (ocd) & anxiety = take st. John's wort, make a tea from dried st. John's wort flowers or consume st. John's wort supplements to help manage ocd. Dosage: drink 1 cup of st. John's wort tea 1-2 times daily or

follow supplement dosage recommendations.

585. Oral thrush = take coconut oil, swish coconut oil in the mouth for a few minutes to help manage oral thrush. Dosage: swish 1 tablespoon of coconut oil in the mouth for 5-10 minutes daily.

586. Osteoarthritis = take ginger, use ginger in cooking or make a tea from fresh ginger to reduce inflammation associated with osteoarthritis. Dosage: use ginger in cooking regularly or drink 1-2 cups of ginger tea daily.

587. Osteoarthritis & joint degeneration = take turmeric, use turmeric powder in cooking or make a tea with turmeric and black pepper to help manage osteoarthritis. Dosage: use 1-3 grams of turmeric powder daily in cooking or drink 1-2 cups of turmeric tea daily.

588. Osteomalacia = take vitamin D supplements, consume vitamin D supplements to help manage osteomalacia. Dosage: take 600-800 iu of vitamin D daily, or follow healthcare provider's recommendations based on blood levels.

589. Osteomalacia & soft bones = take vitamin D, consume vitamin D-rich foods or supplements to help support bone health. Dosage: take 600-800 iu of vitamin D daily, or follow healthcare provider's recommendations based on blood levels.

590. Osteomyelitis & bone infection = take echinacea, consume echinacea supplements or make a tea from dried echinacea to help boost the immune system and manage osteomyelitis. Dosage: drink 1 cup of echinacea tea 1-2 times daily or follow supplement dosage recommendations.

591. Osteoporosis = take red clover, make a tea from dried red clover flowers to support bone health and potentially reduce osteoporosis risk. Dosage: drink 1-2 cups of red clover tea daily.

592. Otitis media = take garlic, apply garlic-infused oil as ear drops to help manage otitis media. Dosage: use garlic-infused oil

as ear drops 2-3 drops in the affected ear twice daily.

593. Ovarian cysts & polycystic ovary syndrome (pcos) = take chasteberry, make a tea from dried chasteberry or consume chasteberry supplements to help manage ovarian cysts. Dosage: drink 1 cup of chasteberry tea daily or follow supplement dosage recommendations.

594. Painful periods & dysmenorrhea = take ginger, make a tea from fresh ginger to help alleviate menstrual cramps. Dosage: drink 1-2 cups of ginger tea daily during menstruation, or as needed for pain relief.

595. Pancreatitis = take turmeric, use turmeric powder in cooking or make a tea with turmeric and black pepper for anti-inflammatory effects to help manage pancreatitis. Dosage: use 1-3 grams of turmeric powder daily in cooking or drink 1-2 cups of turmeric tea daily.

596. Pancreatitis & pancreas inflammation = take licorice root, make a tea from dried licorice root to help soothe and support the pancreas. Dosage: drink 1-2 cups of licorice root tea daily.

597. Parkinson's disease & movement disorder = take mucuna pruriens, consume mucuna pruriens supplements to help support dopamine levels and manage parkinson's symptoms. Dosage: take 100-200 mg of mucuna pruriens supplements daily, or follow healthcare provider's recommendations.

598. Parkinson's disease & tremors = take mucuna pruriens, consume mucuna pruriens supplements to help support motor function in parkinson's disease. Dosage: take 100-200 mg of mucuna pruriens supplements daily, or follow healthcare provider's recommendations.

599. Paroxysmal nocturnal hemoglobinuria (PNH) = consume turmeric to reduce inflammation. Dosage: take 400-600 mg of curcumin supplements 2-3 times daily.

600. Peptic ulcer = take cabbage juice, drink fresh cabbage juice to help soothe peptic ulcers. Dosage: drink 1-2 cups of fresh cabbage juice daily on an empty stomach.

601. Peptic ulcers & stomach ulcers = take cabbage juice, drink fresh cabbage juice to help manage peptic ulcers. Dosage: drink 1-2 cups of fresh cabbage juice daily on an empty stomach.

602. Peripheral neuropathy & nerve damage = take alpha-lipoic acid, consume alpha-lipoic acid supplements to help support nerve health. Dosage: take 600-1200 mg of alpha-lipoic acid daily, or follow healthcare provider's recommendations.

603. Pharyngitis = take marshmallow root, steep dried marshmallow root in hot water for 10 minutes to make a soothing tea for pharyngitis. Dosage: drink 1 cup of marshmallow root tea 1-3 times daily as needed for sore throat relief.

604. Pharyngitis & sore throat = take marshmallow root, make a tea from dried marshmallow root to help soothe a sore throat. Dosage: drink 1 cup of marshmallow root tea 1-3 times daily as needed for sore throat relief.

605. Photophobia = take bilberry, consume bilberry supplements or make a tea from dried bilberry leaves to help manage photophobia. Dosage: drink 1 cup of bilberry tea daily or follow supplement dosage recommendations.

606. Pinworms = take wormwood, consume wormwood supplements or make a tea from dried wormwood leaves to help manage pinworms. Dosage: drink 1 cup of wormwood tea daily or follow supplement dosage recommendations.

607. Plantar fasciitis = take turmeric, use turmeric powder in cooking or make a tea with turmeric and black pepper for anti-inflammatory effects to help manage plantar fasciitis. Dosage: use 1-3 grams of turmeric powder daily in cooking or drink 1-2 cups of turmeric tea daily.

608. Plantar fasciitis & heel pain = take turmeric, use turmeric powder in cooking or make a tea with turmeric and black pepper to help manage inflammation. Dosage: use 1-3 grams of turmeric powder daily in cooking or drink 1-2 cups of turmeric tea daily.

609. Pleurisy & chest pain = take mullein, make a tea from dried mullein leaves to help manage pleurisy. Dosage: drink 1 cup of mullein tea 1-3 times daily as needed for chest pain relief.

610. Pms (premenstrual syndrome) = take chasteberry (vitex), consume chasteberry supplements or make a tea from dried chasteberry fruit to alleviate pms symptoms. Dosage: drink 1 cup of chasteberry tea daily or follow supplement dosage recommendations.

611. Pneumonia = take garlic, consume raw garlic or garlic supplements to support immune function and help manage pneumonia. Dosage: eat 1-2 cloves of raw garlic daily or follow supplement dosage recommendations.

612. Pneumonia & lung infection = take elecampane, make a tea from dried elecampane root to help support lung health. Dosage: drink 1 cup of elecampane tea 1-3 times daily during respiratory infections.

613. Poison ivy & skin rash = take jewelweed, apply jewelweed sap directly to the affected areas to help manage poison ivy rash. Dosage: apply jewelweed sap as needed directly to affected skin.

614. Polycystic kidney disease & kidney cysts = take nettle, make a tea from dried nettle leaves or consume nettle supplements to help support kidney health. Dosage: drink 1-2 cups of nettle tea daily or follow supplement dosage recommendations.

615. Poor circulation = take cayenne pepper, consume cayenne pepper in food or make a tea from dried cayenne pepper to improve circulation. Dosage: add a pinch of cayenne pepper to food daily or drink 1 cup of cayenne tea 1-2 times daily.

616. Postpartum depression = take lemon balm, make a tea from dried lemon balm leaves to help alleviate symptoms of postpartum depression. Dosage: drink 1-2 cups of lemon balm tea daily, or as needed for mood support.

617. Premature ejaculation = take ginkgo biloba, make a tea from dried ginkgo

biloba leaves or consume ginkgo biloba supplements to help manage premature ejaculation. Dosage: drink 1 cup of ginkgo biloba tea daily or follow supplement dosage recommendations.

618. Primary biliary cholangitis = take burdock root to support liver function. Dosage: drink 1 cup of burdock root tea 2-3 times daily or take 500-1,000 mg of burdock root extract daily.

619. Primary sclerosing cholangitis (PSC) = use dandelion root for liver support. Dosage: drink 1-2 cups of dandelion root tea daily or take 1-2 grams of dandelion root powder per day.

620. Prostate problems = take saw palmetto, consume saw palmetto supplements or make a tea from dried saw palmetto berries to support prostate health. Dosage: take 320 mg of saw palmetto extract daily, or follow supplement dosage recommendations.

621. Prostatitis & prostate inflammation = take saw palmetto, consume saw palmetto supplements to help manage prostatitis. Dosage: take 320 mg of saw palmetto extract daily, or follow supplement dosage recommendations.

622. Pruritus = take oatmeal, apply colloidal oatmeal to affected areas to help soothe pruritus (itching). Dosage: apply colloidal oatmeal paste to affected skin 1-2 times daily, or take oatmeal baths as needed.

623. Pulmonary arterial hypertension (PAH) = use ginkgo biloba to improve circulation. Dosage: take 120-240 mg of ginkgo biloba extract daily, divided into two or three doses.

624. Pulmonary embolism = consume ginger to reduce blood clotting. Dosage: drink 1-2 cups of ginger tea daily or take 500-1,000 mg of ginger supplements 2-3 times daily.

625. Pulmonary embolism & lung blood clot = take ginger, make a tea from fresh ginger to help support blood circulation and reduce the risk of clots. Dosage: drink 1-2 cups of ginger tea daily.

626. Pyelonephritis = take cranberry, drink cranberry juice or consume dried

cranberries to help manage pyelonephritis. Dosage: drink 8-16 ounces of cranberry juice daily, or follow supplement dosage recommendations.

627. Pyelonephritis & kidney infection = take cranberry, consume cranberry juice or supplements to help manage kidney infections. Dosage: drink 8-16 ounces of cranberry juice daily, or follow supplement dosage recommendations.

628. Radiation exposure = take spirulina, consume spirulina supplements to help detoxify the body from radiation exposure. Dosage: take 1-2 teaspoons of spirulina powder daily, or follow supplement dosage recommendations.

629. Rash = take chamomile, apply chamomile cream or make a tea from dried chamomile flowers to soothe skin rash. Dosage: apply chamomile cream to affected skin 1-3 times daily or drink 1-2 cups of chamomile tea daily.

630. Raynaud's disease & poor circulation = take ginger, make a tea from fresh ginger to help improve circulation. Dosage: drink 1-2 cups of ginger tea daily.

631. Respiratory issues = take thyme, brew leaves in hot water or inhale steam from hot water infused with thyme for respiratory issues. Dosage: drink 1-2 cups of thyme tea daily, or inhale steam for 10-15 minutes as needed.

632. Restless leg syndrome (rls) = take iron, consume iron-rich foods or supplements to help alleviate symptoms of restless leg syndrome. Dosage: consume 18 mg of iron daily, or follow healthcare provider's recommendations.

633. Restless legs syndrome (rls) & leg discomfort = take magnesium, consume magnesium-rich foods or supplements to help manage rls. Dosage: take 400-500 mg of magnesium daily, or follow healthcare provider's recommendations.

634. Retinal detachment & vision loss = take bilberry, consume bilberry supplements or make a tea from dried bilberry leaves to support eye health. Dosage: drink 1-2

cups of bilberry tea daily, or follow supplement dosage recommendations.

635. Rheumatic fever & inflammatory disease = take willow bark, make a tea from dried willow bark to help reduce inflammation and manage pain associated with rheumatic fever. Dosage: drink 1-2 cups of willow bark tea daily.

636. Rheumatic heart disease = take garlic for its cardiovascular benefits. Dosage: consume 1-2 cloves of raw garlic daily or take 600-1,200 mg of garlic supplements daily.

637. Rheumatoid arthritis = take turmeric, use turmeric powder in cooking or make a tea with turmeric and black pepper for anti-inflammatory effects. Dosage: use 1-3 grams of turmeric powder daily in cooking or drink 1-2 cups of turmeric tea daily.

638. Rickets = take vitamin D supplements, consume vitamin D supplements to help manage rickets. Dosage: take 600-800 iu of vitamin D daily, or follow healthcare provider's recommendations based on blood levels.

639. Ringworm = take garlic, apply crushed garlic directly to affected areas to treat ringworm. Dosage: apply crushed garlic to affected skin for 10-15 minutes, then rinse. Repeat 2-3 times daily.

640. Rosacea = take green tea, make a tea from dried green tea leaves or use green tea extract topically to help manage rosacea. Dosage: drink 1-2 cups of green tea daily, or apply green tea extract to affected areas as directed.

641. Rosacea & facial redness = take chamomile, make a tea from dried chamomile flowers and use as a facial wash to help manage rosacea. Dosage: use chamomile tea as a facial wash 1-2 times daily, or drink 1-2 cups of chamomile tea daily.

642. Salivary gland stones = Take lemon juice, consume freshly squeezed lemon juice diluted with water to help stimulate saliva flow and dislodge stones. Dosage: 1-2

tablespoons in a glass of water, 2-3 times daily.

643. Sarcoidosis = take turmeric, use turmeric powder in cooking or make a tea with turmeric and black pepper for anti-inflammatory effects to help manage sarcoidosis. Dosage: use 1-2 grams of turmeric powder daily in cooking, or drink 1-2 cups of turmeric tea daily.

644. Scabies & skin mites = take neem oil, apply neem oil to the affected areas to help manage scabies. Dosage: apply neem oil to affected skin 1-2 times daily.

645. Scarlet fever = Take echinacea, make a tea from dried echinacea or consume echinacea supplements to help support the immune system. Dosage: 1-2 cups of tea daily or 300 mg of supplement, 3 times daily.

646. Schistosomiasis (bilharzia) = Take garlic, consume raw garlic or garlic supplements to help fight the infection. Dosage: 1-2 raw garlic cloves daily or 600-1200 mg of aged garlic extract daily.

647. Schizophrenia = take ginkgo biloba, make a tea from dried ginkgo biloba leaves or consume ginkgo biloba supplements to potentially benefit cognitive function in schizophrenia. Dosage: drink 1-2 cups of ginkgo biloba tea daily, or follow supplement dosage recommendations.

648. Sciatica = take devil's claw, make a tea from dried devil's claw root to help alleviate sciatica pain. Dosage: drink 1-2 cups of devil's claw tea daily.

649. Scleroderma = Take evening primrose oil, consume evening primrose oil supplements to help manage skin symptoms and inflammation. Dosage: 500 mg, 2-3 times daily.

650. Scleroderma & skin hardening = take gotu kola, consume gotu kola supplements to help support skin health. Dosage: take 500 mg of gotu kola supplements 1-2 times daily, or follow healthcare provider's recommendations.

651. Scoliosis = Take turmeric, use turmeric powder in cooking, or make a tea with turmeric and black pepper to help manage

inflammation. Dosage: 1 teaspoon of turmeric powder with a pinch of black pepper in a cup of hot water, 1-2 times daily.

652.Scurvy = take citrus fruits, consume citrus fruits such as oranges and lemons to help manage scurvy. Dosage: consume 1-2 servings of citrus fruits daily.

653.Seasonal affective disorder (SAD) = Take St. John's Wort, make a tea from dried St. John's Wort or consume St. John's Wort supplements to help manage SAD. Dosage: 300 mg of extract, 3 times daily.

654.Seborrheic dermatitis & scalp itching = take tea tree oil, use a shampoo with tea tree oil or apply diluted tea tree oil to the scalp to help manage seborrheic dermatitis. Dosage: use tea tree oil shampoo as directed, or apply diluted tea tree oil to scalp 1-2 times weekly.

655.Seizures = take lavender, use lavender essential oil in aromatherapy or make a tea from dried lavender flowers to help manage seizures. Dosage: inhale lavender essential oil from a diffuser, or drink 1 cup of lavender tea daily.

656.Sepsis = Take echinacea, make a tea from dried echinacea or consume echinacea supplements to help support the immune system. Dosage: 1-2 cups of tea daily or 300 mg of supplement, 3 times daily.

657.Sepsis & blood infection = take echinacea, make a tea from dried echinacea or consume echinacea supplements to help support the immune system and manage sepsis. Dosage: drink 1-2 cups of echinacea tea daily, or follow supplement dosage recommendations.

658.Septic arthritis = Take turmeric, use turmeric powder in cooking or make a tea with turmeric and black pepper to help manage inflammation. Dosage: 1 teaspoon of turmeric powder with a pinch of black pepper in a cup of hot water, 1-2 times daily.

659.Septicaemia = Take echinacea, make a tea from dried echinacea or consume echinacea supplements to help support the immune system. Dosage: 1-2 cups of tea daily or 300 mg of supplement, 3 times daily.

660. Sexual dysfunction = take ginseng, consume ginseng root or make a tea to help manage sexual dysfunction. Dosage: drink 1-2 cups of ginseng tea daily, or follow supplement dosage recommendations.

661. Shin splints = take turmeric, use turmeric powder in cooking or make a tea with turmeric and black pepper for anti-inflammatory effects to help manage shin splints. Dosage: use 1-2 grams of turmeric powder daily in cooking, or drink 1-2 cups of turmeric tea daily.

662. Shingles = take lemon balm, apply lemon balm cream or ointment to shingles blisters for soothing relief. Dosage: apply lemon balm cream to affected areas 2-3 times daily.

663. Shoulder pain = take ginger, chew raw ginger or make a tea from fresh ginger slices to help manage shoulder pain. Dosage: chew 1-2 slices of fresh ginger daily, or drink 1-2 cups of ginger tea daily.

664. Sickle cell disease = take papaya leaf extract, consume papaya leaf extract to help manage symptoms of sickle cell disease. Dosage: follow papaya leaf extract supplement dosage recommendations.

665. Sinus headaches = take feverfew, consume fresh leaves or make a tea with dried feverfew leaves to help manage sinus headaches. Dosage: drink 1-2 cups of feverfew tea daily.

666. Sinusitis = take eucalyptus, use eucalyptus oil in steam inhalation or make a tea from dried eucalyptus leaves to help manage sinusitis. Dosage: inhale eucalyptus steam for 10-15 minutes 1-2 times daily, or drink 1-2 cups of eucalyptus tea daily.

667. Sjogren's syndrome = use aloe vera to relieve dry mouth and eyes. Dosage: drink 1/4 cup of aloe vera juice daily or apply aloe vera gel to affected areas as needed.

668. Sjogren's syndrome & dryness = take slippery elm, make a tea from dried slippery elm bark or consume slippery elm supplements to help manage dryness.

Dosage: drink 1 cup of slippery elm tea 1-3 times daily.

669. Skin infections and acne = take tea tree oil, dilute with a carrier oil and apply to skin infections and acne. Dosage: apply diluted tea tree oil to affected areas 1-2 times daily.

670. Skin tags & benign growths = take tea tree oil, apply diluted tea tree oil to the skin tags to help remove them. Dosage: apply diluted tea tree oil to skin tags 1-2 times daily until they fall off.

671. Sleep apnea = take valerian root, steep dried valerian root in hot water for 10-15 minutes to make a tea to help manage sleep apnea. Dosage: drink 1 cup of valerian root tea 30 minutes before bedtime.

672. Sleepwalking = take valerian root, steep dried valerian root in hot water for 10-15 minutes to make a tea to help manage sleepwalking. Dosage: drink 1 cup of valerian root tea 30 minutes before bedtime.

673. Snake bites = Take echinacea, make a tea from dried echinacea or consume echinacea supplements to help support the immune system. Dosage: 1-2 cups of tea daily or 300 mg of supplement, 3 times daily.

674. Snoring = take peppermint, make a tea from dried peppermint leaves or use peppermint essential oil in aromatherapy to help reduce snoring. Dosage: drink 1 cup of peppermint tea before bedtime, or use peppermint essential oil in a diffuser.

675. Sore nipples & breastfeeding pain = take calendula, apply calendula ointment to the affected areas to help soothe sore nipples. Dosage: apply calendula ointment to sore nipples 1-2 times daily.

676. Sore throat = take marshmallow root, make a tea from dried marshmallow root or use marshmallow root lozenges to help soothe the sore throat. Dosage: drink 1-2 cups of marshmallow root tea daily, or use lozenges as needed.

677. Sore throats and coughs = take honey, take a spoonful or mix with warm water

and lemon for sore throats and coughs. Dosage: take 1-2 tablespoons of honey daily.

678. Sore throats and digestive issues = take slippery elm, mix powdered bark with hot water to make a soothing tea for sore throats and digestive issues. Dosage: drink 1 cup of slippery elm tea 1-3 times daily.

679. Speech disorders = take ginkgo biloba, make a tea from dried ginkgo biloba leaves or consume ginkgo biloba supplements to potentially benefit cognitive function and help manage speech disorders. Dosage: drink 1-2 cups of ginkgo biloba tea daily, or follow supplement dosage recommendations.

680. Sperm count (low) = Take ashwagandha, consume ashwagandha supplements to help increase sperm count. Dosage: 600 mg of extract daily.

681. Spider bites = take witch hazel, apply witch hazel directly to spider bites to help reduce inflammation and soothe itching.

Dosage: apply witch hazel to the affected area 2-3 times daily.

682. Spina bifida = Take folic acid, consume folic acid supplements to help manage spina bifida. Dosage: 400-800 mcg daily.

683. Spinal cord injury & spinal damage = take turmeric, use turmeric powder in cooking or make a tea with turmeric and black pepper to help manage inflammation and support healing in spinal cord injury. Dosage: use 1-2 grams of turmeric powder daily in cooking, or drink 1-2 cups of turmeric tea daily.

684. Spinal muscular atrophy = Take coenzyme Q10, consume CoQ10 supplements to help support muscle function. Dosage: 200 mg daily.

685. Spirometry = No specific herbal remedy. Spirometry is a diagnostic test to measure lung function.

686. Spleen problems and spleen removal = Take milk thistle, make a tea from dried milk thistle or consume milk thistle supplements to help support liver function and compensate for spleen

removal. Dosage: 200-400 mg of extract daily.

687. Spondylolisthesis = Take turmeric, use turmeric powder in cooking or make a tea with turmeric and black pepper to help manage inflammation. Dosage: 1 teaspoon of turmeric powder with a pinch of black pepper in a cup of hot water, 1-2 times daily.

688. Sprains = take arnica, apply arnica cream or gel to affected area to help reduce inflammation and pain in sprains. Dosage: apply arnica cream or gel to the affected area 2-3 times daily.

689. Sprains & ligament injuries = take arnica, apply arnica cream to the affected areas to help reduce inflammation and pain. Dosage: apply arnica cream to affected areas 2-3 times daily.

690. Sprains and strains = Take arnica, apply arnica cream or gel to the affected area to help reduce inflammation and pain. Dosage: Apply 2-3 times daily.

691. Squint = Take bilberry, consume bilberry supplements or make a tea from dried bilberry leaves to support eye health. Dosage: 160 mg of extract daily or 1-2 cups of tea daily.

692. Staph infection & bacterial infection = take garlic, consume raw garlic or garlic supplements to help fight staph infections. Dosage: consume 1-2 cloves of raw garlic daily or follow supplement dosage recommendations.

693. Stomach cancer & gastric cancer = take green tea, drink green tea regularly to help support overall health and manage stomach cancer. Dosage: drink 2-3 cups of green tea daily.

694. Stomach ulcer = take cabbage juice, drink fresh cabbage juice to help soothe stomach ulcers. Dosage: drink 1/2 cup of fresh cabbage juice 2-3 times daily.

695. Stress = take ashwagandha, consume ashwagandha supplements or make a tea from dried ashwagandha root to reduce stress levels. Dosage: drink 1 cup of ashwagandha tea daily, or follow supplement dosage recommendations.

696. Stress and energy = take ashwagandha, brew root powder in hot water for 10 minutes or take in supplement form to reduce stress and boost energy. Dosage: drink 1 cup of ashwagandha tea daily, or follow supplement dosage recommendations.

697. Stress and sleep = take lavender, brew flowers in hot water or use essential oil in a diffuser to relieve stress and improve sleep. Dosage: drink 1 cup of lavender tea before bedtime, or diffuse lavender essential oil for 30-60 minutes.

698. Stretch marks = Take gotu kola, apply gotu kola cream to the affected area to help reduce the appearance of stretch marks. Dosage: Apply 2-3 times daily.

699. Stroke = Take ginkgo biloba, make a tea from dried ginkgo biloba leaves or consume ginkgo biloba supplements to help improve blood circulation and brain function. Dosage: 120-240 mg of extract daily or 1-2 cups of tea daily.

700. Stroke prevention & brain health = take ginkgo biloba, make a tea from dried ginkgo biloba leaves or consume ginkgo biloba supplements to support brain health. Dosage: drink 1-2 cups of ginkgo biloba tea daily, or follow supplement dosage recommendations.

701. Stuttering = take passionflower, make a tea from dried passionflower leaves and flowers to help reduce stuttering. Dosage: drink 1 cup of passionflower tea daily.

702. Stye & eye infection = take chamomile, make a tea from dried chamomile flowers and use as a compress to help manage styes. Dosage: apply chamomile tea compress to the affected eye for 10-15 minutes, 2-3 times daily.

703. Sunburn & skin damage = take aloe vera, apply aloe vera gel to the affected areas to help soothe sunburn. Dosage: apply aloe vera gel to sunburned skin as needed.

704. Sweating (excessive) = take sage, make a tea from dried sage leaves or use sage essential oil in aromatherapy to help manage excessive sweating. Dosage: drink 1 cup of sage tea daily, or use sage essential oil in a diffuser.

705. Swimmer's ear & ear infection = take garlic oil, apply garlic oil drops in the ear to help manage swimmer's ear. Dosage: apply 2-3 drops of garlic oil into the affected ear 1-2 times daily.

706. Swollen eyelids = take chamomile, make a tea from dried chamomile flowers or use chamomile-infused eye drops to help reduce swelling in eyelids. Dosage: apply chamomile tea compress to the affected eyelid for 10-15 minutes, 2-3 times daily.

707. Swollen feet and ankles = take dandelion, make a tea from dried dandelion leaves or consume dandelion supplements to help reduce swelling in feet and ankles. Dosage: drink 1-2 cups of dandelion tea daily, or follow supplement dosage recommendations.

708. Swollen glands = take echinacea, consume echinacea supplements or make a tea from dried echinacea roots to help manage swollen glands. Dosage: drink 1-2 cups of echinacea tea daily, or follow supplement dosage recommendations.

709. Swollen lymph nodes & lymphadenopathy = take cleavers, make a tea from dried cleavers leaves to help reduce swollen lymph nodes. Dosage: drink 1-2 cups of cleavers tea daily.

710. Syphilis & sexually transmitted infection = take sarsaparilla, make a tea from dried sarsaparilla root to help manage syphilis. Dosage: drink 1-2 cups of sarsaparilla tea daily.

711. Systemic lupus erythematosus (sle) = take turmeric, use turmeric powder in cooking or make a tea with turmeric and black pepper for anti-inflammatory effects in sle. Dosage: use 1-2 grams of turmeric powder daily in cooking, or drink 1-2 cups of turmeric tea daily.

712. Systemic lupus erythematosus (sle) & autoimmune disease = take reishi mushroom, consume reishi mushroom supplements to help support immune function and manage sle. Dosage: follow reishi mushroom supplement dosage recommendations.

713.Tachycardia = take hawthorn, make a tea from dried hawthorn berries or consume hawthorn supplements to help manage tachycardia. Dosage: drink 1-2 cups of hawthorn tea daily, or follow supplement dosage recommendations.

714.Takayasu's arteritis = take omega-3 fatty acids to reduce inflammation. Dosage: take 1,000-3,000 mg of omega-3 supplements daily.

715.Tapeworms = take wormwood, consume wormwood supplements or make a tea from dried wormwood leaves to help manage tapeworms. Dosage: drink 1 cup of wormwood tea daily, or follow supplement dosage recommendations.

716.Teething pain = take chamomile, make a tea from dried chamomile flowers to help soothe teething pain. Dosage: give 1-2 teaspoons of cooled chamomile tea to the infant as needed.

717.Telogen effluvium = take saw palmetto, consume saw palmetto supplements or apply saw palmetto extract to the scalp to support hair growth in telogen effluvium. Dosage: follow saw palmetto supplement dosage recommendations, or apply saw palmetto extract to the scalp once daily.

718.Temporal arteritis = take turmeric, use turmeric powder in cooking or make a tea with turmeric and black pepper for anti-inflammatory effects to help manage temporal arteritis. Dosage: use 1-2 grams of turmeric powder daily in cooking, or drink 1-2 cups of turmeric tea daily.

719.Tendinitis = take arnica, apply arnica cream or gel to affected area to help reduce inflammation and pain in tendinitis. Dosage: apply arnica cream or gel to the affected area 2-3 times daily.

720.Tendinitis & tendon inflammation = take turmeric, use turmeric powder in cooking or make a tea with turmeric and black pepper to help manage tendinitis. Dosage: use 1-2 grams of turmeric powder daily in cooking, or drink 1-2 cups of turmeric tea daily.

721.Tennis elbow = take turmeric, use turmeric powder in cooking or make a tea with turmeric and black pepper for anti-inflammatory effects to help manage tennis elbow. Dosage: use 1-2 grams of turmeric powder daily in cooking, or drink 1-2 cups of turmeric tea daily.

722. Tension headaches & stress = take feverfew, make a tea from dried feverfew leaves or consume feverfew supplements to help manage tension headaches. Dosage: drink 1 cup of feverfew tea daily, or follow supplement dosage recommendations.

723. Testicular pain = take ginger, chew raw ginger or make a tea from fresh ginger slices to help manage testicular pain. Dosage: chew 1-2 slices of fresh ginger daily, or drink 1-2 cups of ginger tea daily.

724. Testicular pain & epididymitis = take saw palmetto, consume saw palmetto supplements to help manage testicular pain. Dosage: follow saw palmetto supplement dosage recommendations.

725. Tetanus = take echinacea, consume echinacea supplements or make a tea from dried echinacea roots to support immune function in tetanus. Dosage:

drink 1-2 cups of echinacea tea daily, or follow supplement dosage recommendations.

726. Thalassemia = consume spirulina to support red blood cell production. Dosage: take 1-3 grams of spirulina powder daily or as directed on the supplement label.

727. Thalassemia & blood disorder = take spirulina, consume spirulina supplements to help support red blood cell production in thalassemia. Dosage: follow spirulina supplement dosage recommendations.

728. Throat cancer & tumors = take green tea, drink green tea regularly to provide antioxidant support to help manage throat cancer. Dosage: drink 2-3 cups of green tea daily.

729. Thrombocytopenia = take papaya leaf extract, consume papaya leaf extract to help increase platelet count in thrombocytopenia. Dosage: follow papaya leaf extract supplement dosage recommendations.

730. Thrombocytopenia & low platelet count = take papaya leaf, make a tea from papaya leaves to help increase platelet count. Dosage: drink 1-2 cups of papaya leaf tea daily.

731. Thrombosis & blood clot = take nattokinase, consume nattokinase supplements to help support blood flow and reduce clot formation. Dosage: follow nattokinase supplement dosage recommendations.

732. Thrush = take coconut oil, swish coconut oil in the mouth for a few minutes or apply topically to help manage thrush. Dosage: swish 1 tablespoon of coconut oil in the mouth for 5-10 minutes daily.

733. Thyroid cancer & thyroid tumor = take bladderwrack, consume bladderwrack supplements to help support thyroid health. Dosage: follow bladderwrack supplement dosage recommendations.

734. Thyroid nodules & swelling = take ashwagandha, consume ashwagandha supplements to help manage thyroid nodules. Dosage: follow ashwagandha supplement dosage recommendations.

735. Tinea cruris = take tea tree oil, apply diluted tea tree oil directly to affected areas to treat tinea cruris. Dosage: apply diluted tea tree oil to the affected area 2-3 times daily.

736. Tinea versicolor = take apple cider vinegar, apply diluted apple cider vinegar topically to affected areas to help manage tinea versicolor. Dosage: apply diluted apple cider vinegar to the affected area once daily.

737. Tinnitus = take ginkgo biloba, make a tea from dried ginkgo biloba leaves or consume ginkgo biloba supplements to alleviate tinnitus symptoms. Dosage: drink 1-2 cups of ginkgo biloba tea daily, or follow supplement dosage recommendations.

738. Tinnitus & ringing ears = take ginkgo biloba, make a tea from dried ginkgo biloba leaves or consume ginkgo biloba supplements to help manage tinnitus. Dosage: drink 1-2 cups of ginkgo biloba

tea daily, or follow supplement dosage recommendations.

739. Toenail fungus = take tea tree oil, apply diluted tea tree oil directly to affected toenails to help manage toenail fungus. Dosage: apply diluted tea tree oil to the affected toenail 2-3 times daily.

740. Tonsillitis = take slippery elm, make a tea from dried slippery elm bark or consume slippery elm supplements to help soothe tonsillitis symptoms. Dosage: drink 1-2 cups of slippery elm tea daily, or follow supplement dosage recommendations.

741. Tonsillitis & throat infection = take echinacea, make a tea from dried echinacea or consume echinacea supplements to help manage tonsillitis. Dosage: drink 1-2 cups of echinacea tea daily, or follow supplement dosage recommendations.

742. Toothache = take clove, apply clove oil to the affected area or chew on a whole clove for toothache relief. Dosage: apply clove oil to the affected area 2-3 times daily, or chew on a whole clove as needed.

743. Tourette syndrome & neurological disorder = take passionflower, make a tea from dried passionflower to help manage tics and anxiety in tourette syndrome. Dosage: drink 1 cup of passionflower tea daily.

744. Toxemia & blood poisoning = take burdock root, make a tea from dried burdock root to help detoxify the blood. Dosage: drink 1-2 cups of burdock root tea daily.

745. Toxoplasmosis = take garlic, consume raw garlic or garlic supplements to help combat toxoplasmosis. Dosage: consume 2-3 cloves of raw garlic daily, or follow supplement dosage recommendations.

746. Trichomoniasis = take goldenseal, consume goldenseal supplements or make a tea from dried goldenseal root to help manage trichomoniasis. Dosage: drink 1-2 cups of goldenseal tea daily, or follow supplement dosage recommendations.

747. Trichomoniasis & parasitic infection = take goldenseal, make a tea from dried

goldenseal root or consume goldenseal supplements to help manage trichomoniasis. Dosage: drink 1-2 cups of goldenseal tea daily, or follow supplement dosage recommendations.

748. Trigeminal neuralgia = use capsaicin to relieve nerve pain. Dosage: apply capsaicin cream to the affected area 2-3 times daily.

749. Trigeminal neuralgia & facial nerve pain = take st. John's wort, make a tea from dried st. John's wort flowers to help manage nerve pain. Dosage: drink 1-2 cups of st. John's wort tea daily.

750. Trigeminal neuralgia & facial pain = take skullcap, make a tea from dried skullcap leaves to help manage trigeminal neuralgia. Dosage: drink 1-2 cups of skullcap tea daily.

751. Tuberculosis (tb) = take garlic, consume raw garlic or garlic supplements to potentially benefit respiratory health and help manage tuberculosis. Dosage: consume 2-3 cloves of raw garlic daily, or follow supplement dosage recommendations.

752. Tuberculosis & bacterial infection = take garlic, consume raw garlic or garlic supplements to help support the immune system and manage tuberculosis. Dosage: consume 2-3 cloves of raw garlic daily, or follow supplement dosage recommendations.

753. Typhoid fever = take neem, consume neem leaves or neem supplements to help manage symptoms of typhoid fever. Dosage: drink neem tea made from fresh or dried leaves 1-2 times daily, or follow supplement dosage recommendations.

754. Ulcerative colitis = take slippery elm, consume slippery elm supplements or make a tea from dried slippery elm bark to help soothe ulcerative colitis symptoms. Dosage: drink 1-2 cups of slippery elm tea daily, or follow supplement dosage recommendations.

755. Ulcerative colitis & inflammatory bowel disease = take slippery elm, make a tea from dried slippery elm bark to help

soothe the digestive tract in ulcerative colitis. Dosage: drink 1-2 cups of slippery elm tea daily.

756. Ulcerative colitis & intestinal inflammation = take aloe vera, consume aloe vera juice to help manage ulcerative colitis. Dosage: drink 1/2 cup of aloe vera juice daily.

757. Umbilical hernia = take ginger, chew raw ginger or make a tea from fresh ginger slices to alleviate umbilical hernia symptoms. Dosage: chew 1-2 slices of fresh ginger daily, or drink 1-2 cups of ginger tea daily.

758. Urinary incontinence = take pumpkin seed extract, consume pumpkin seed extract to help alleviate urinary incontinence. Dosage: follow pumpkin seed extract supplement dosage recommendations.

759. Urinary tract infection (uti) = take cranberry, drink cranberry juice or consume dried cranberries to prevent and treat utis. Dosage: drink 1-2 cups of cranberry juice daily, or consume a handful of dried cranberries daily.

760. Uterine fibroids & noncancerous tumors = take chasteberry, make a tea from dried chasteberry or consume chasteberry supplements to help manage uterine fibroids. Dosage: drink 1-2 cups of chasteberry tea daily, or follow supplement dosage recommendations.

761. Uterine fibroids & uterine tumors = take chasteberry, consume chasteberry supplements to help manage symptoms of uterine fibroids. Dosage: follow chasteberry supplement dosage recommendations.

762. Varicella = take chamomile, apply chamomile cream or make a tea from dried chamomile flowers to soothe varicella symptoms. Dosage: drink 1-2 cups of chamomile tea daily, or apply chamomile cream as needed.

763. Varicose veins = take horse chestnut, apply horse chestnut cream to affected areas to reduce varicose veins. Dosage:

apply horse chestnut cream to the affected area 2-3 times daily.

764. Varicose veins & venous disorder = take horse chestnut, apply horse chestnut cream or consume horse chestnut supplements to help manage varicose veins. Dosage: apply horse chestnut cream to the affected area 2-3 times daily, or follow supplement dosage recommendations.

765. Vasculitis & blood vessel inflammation = take turmeric, use turmeric powder in cooking or make a tea with turmeric and black pepper to help manage vasculitis. Dosage: use 1-2 grams of turmeric powder daily in cooking, or drink 1-2 cups of turmeric tea daily.

766. Vertebral subluxation = take turmeric, use turmeric powder in cooking or make a tea with turmeric and black pepper for anti-inflammatory effects to help manage vertebral subluxation. Dosage: use 1-2 grams of turmeric powder daily in cooking, or drink 1-2 cups of turmeric tea daily.

767. Vertigo = take ginger, chew raw ginger or make a tea from fresh ginger slices to alleviate vertigo symptoms. Dosage: chew 1-2 slices of fresh ginger daily, or drink 1-2 cups of ginger tea daily.

768. Viral hepatitis & liver infection = take dandelion root, make a tea from dried dandelion root to help support liver health in viral hepatitis. Dosage: drink 1-2 cups of dandelion root tea daily.

769. Vision loss = take bilberry, consume bilberry supplements or make a tea from dried bilberry leaves to support eye health. Dosage: drink 1-2 cups of bilberry tea daily, or follow supplement dosage recommendations.

770. Vitiligo = take ginkgo biloba, make a tea from dried leaves or consume ginkgo biloba supplements to help manage vitiligo symptoms. Dosage: drink 1-2 cups of ginkgo biloba tea daily, or follow supplement dosage recommendations.

771. Vocal cord nodules & polyps = take licorice root, make a tea from dried licorice root to help soothe the throat and

manage vocal cord nodules. Dosage: drink 1-2 cups of licorice root tea daily.

772. Vomiting = take ginger, chew raw ginger or make a tea from fresh ginger slices to alleviate vomiting. Dosage: chew 1-2 slices of fresh ginger daily, or drink 1-2 cups of ginger tea daily.

773. Von Willebrand disease = Take dong quai, make a tea from dried dong quai to help support blood health. Dosage: 1-2 grams of dried dong quai root per day, steeped in hot water for 10-15 minutes.

774. Von willebrand disease & bleeding disorder = take dong quai, make a tea from dried dong quai to help support blood health. Dosage: drink 1 cup of dong quai tea daily, or follow supplement dosage recommendations.

775. Vulval cancer = Take green tea, drink green tea regularly to provide antioxidant support and potentially help manage vulval cancer. Dosage: 3-4 cups of green tea daily.

776. Water retention & edema = take dandelion, make a tea from dried dandelion leaves or consume dandelion supplements to help reduce water retention. Dosage: drink 1-2 cups of dandelion tea daily, or follow supplement dosage recommendations.

777. Watering eyes = Take eyebright, make a tea from dried eyebright and use it as an eye wash to help manage watering eyes. Dosage: 1 teaspoon of dried eyebright per cup of boiling water, steep for 10 minutes, cool, and use as an eye wash 2-3 times daily.

778. Wegener's granulomatosis (Granulomatosis with polyangiitis) = take boswellia for its anti-inflammatory properties. Dosage: take 300-400 mg of boswellia extract 2-3 times daily.

779. Weight loss = take green tea, steep dried leaves in hot water for 3-5 minutes to aid in weight loss. Dosage: drink 2-3 cups of green tea daily.

780. Wernicke-korsakoff syndrome & neurological disorder = take milk thistle, make a tea from dried milk thistle or consume milk thistle supplements to help

support liver health. Dosage: drink 1-2 cups of milk thistle tea daily, or follow supplement dosage recommendations.

781. West nile virus & mosquito-borne infection = take echinacea, make a tea from dried echinacea or consume echinacea supplements to help support the immune system. Dosage: drink 1-2 cups of echinacea tea daily, or follow supplement dosage recommendations.

782. Whiplash = take arnica, apply arnica cream or gel to affected area to help reduce inflammation and pain. Dosage: apply arnica cream or gel to the affected area 2-3 times daily.

783. Whipple's disease & bacterial infection = take oregano oil, consume oregano oil capsules to help manage whipple's disease. Dosage: follow oregano oil supplement dosage recommendations.

784. Whooping cough & pertussis = take wild cherry bark, make a tea from dried wild cherry bark to help soothe coughs. Dosage: drink 1-2 cups of wild cherry bark tea daily.

785. Wilson's disease & copper accumulation = take milk thistle, make a tea from dried milk thistle or consume milk thistle supplements to help support liver health. Dosage: drink 1-2 cups of milk thistle tea daily, or follow supplement dosage recommendations.

786. Wolff-Parkinson-White syndrome = Take hawthorn, make a tea from dried hawthorn berries or consume hawthorn supplements to help support heart health. Dosage: 160-900 mg of hawthorn extract daily or 1-2 cups of tea.

787. Womb (uterus) cancer = Take green tea, drink green tea regularly to provide antioxidant support and potentially help manage womb cancer. Dosage: 3-4 cups of green tea daily.

788. Wound healing = take comfrey, apply comfrey ointment or poultice to wounds to speed up healing. Dosage: apply comfrey ointment or poultice to the affected area 1-2 times daily.

789. Wounds and inflammation = take comfrey, apply poultices of fresh leaves to

wounds or make a salve for reducing inflammation. Dosage: apply comfrey poultice or salve to the affected area 1-2 times daily.

790. Wrist pain = take turmeric, use turmeric powder in cooking or make a tea with turmeric and black pepper for anti-inflammatory effects to help manage wrist pain. Dosage: use 1-2 grams of turmeric powder daily in cooking, or drink 1-2 cups of turmeric tea daily.

791. Xanthoma = take garlic, consume raw garlic or garlic supplements to help reduce xanthoma. Dosage: 2-3 raw garlic cloves daily or 600-1200 mg garlic supplements.

792. Xerosis = take coconut oil, apply coconut oil topically to dry skin to moisturize and soften. Dosage: apply 2-3 times daily.

793. Xerostomia = take licorice root, chew on licorice root or make a tea from dried licorice root to stimulate saliva production. Dosage: 2-3 cups of tea daily.

794. Yawning = take lavender, use lavender essential oil in aromatherapy to help reduce yawning. Dosage: inhale lavender oil 2-3 times daily.

795. Yeast infection = take garlic, consume raw garlic or garlic supplements to help combat yeast infections. Dosage: 2-3 raw garlic cloves daily or 600-1200 mg garlic supplements.

796. Yeast infection & candidiasis = take tea tree oil, use tea tree oil suppositories or diluted tea tree oil to help manage yeast infections. Dosage: apply topically 2-3 times daily.

797. Yellow fever = take papaya leaf extract, consume papaya leaf extract to help alleviate symptoms of yellow fever. Dosage: 1-2 tablespoons daily.

798. Yellow fever & viral infection = take echinacea, make a tea from dried echinacea or consume echinacea supplements to help support the immune system. Dosage: 300 mg supplements or 1-2 grams dried herb 2-3 times daily.

799. Zenker's diverticulum & throat pouches = take slippery elm, make a tea from dried slippery elm bark or consume slippery elm

supplements to help soothe the throat. Dosage: 1-2 grams dried bark or 400 mg supplements 2-3 times daily.

800. Zika virus = take papaya leaf extract, consume papaya leaf extract to help manage symptoms of zika virus. Dosage: 1-2 tablespoons daily.

801. Zollinger-ellison syndrome & gastric condition = take licorice root, make a tea from dried licorice root to help soothe the digestive tract. Dosage: 1-2 grams dried root 2-3 times daily.

802. Zollinger-ellison syndrome & stomach tumors = take licorice root, make a tea from dried licorice root to help manage stomach acid levels. Dosage: 1-2 grams dried root 2-3 times daily.

803. Zygomycosis & fungal infection = take garlic, consume raw garlic or garlic supplements to help fight fungal infections. Dosage: 2-3 raw garlic cloves daily or 600-1200 mg garlic supplemen

I hope this remedies can be of help to you whenever you need it; herbs are our history; we should not forget them but rather embrace them.

Ailments index with over 800 herbal remedies

BOOK 7:

Detox and Healthy Lifestyle

Detoxifying your life

I love having a cleanse twice a year because it detoxifies my body of all the junk I've been feeding it over the years, which has built up as poisons along my intestinal walls. Your body will benefit greatly from 7 days of solely fruits and vegetables and no coffee, sweets, alcohol, carbohydrates, dairy, or meat. You feel lighter and more invigorated, your digestion is now functioning normally again, and you've probably totally reset your hunger perception and eradicated any cravings. It's a terrific idea to give your body a few days to clear out all the built-up junk and prepare it to face life—and burgers—again.

However, the truth is that poisons are present throughout your entire life, not just in your body. You're constantly getting unsolicited emails, getting notifications on your phone, having clutter in your kitchen, bathroom, and closet, and spending your leisure time with toxic people and unenjoyable activities are all contributing factors to your mental clutter.

Although this may sound a bit dramatic, there's a good probability that you have at least a few bad habits and thought patterns that are detrimental to your mind and spirit, even if you consider yourself to be an extremely successful minimalist.

This is the comprehensive to-do list for detoxing your life in just one week! However, a couple of things before we begin:

It is certainly possible to complete it in less than a week, but I do not advise you to do so. Eliminating various forms of clutter from your life can be a daunting and draining task, and attempting to accomplish it all at once increases the likelihood of giving up. Rather, focus on one area of your life at a time and dedicate enough time to getting it perfect before moving on to the next.

When it is appropriate to do it

A total life detox is an excellent idea at any time because it will clear your mind and provide you with the energy to tackle new challenges. But I discovered that anytime you are going through a change in your life, it's really beneficial to do it at that time: relocating to a new nation. Rather than storing everything in storage, use it as a chance to reduce and get rid of clutter. Obtaining a new job? Give yourself a week to change your perspective and eliminate the negative thought patterns and bad behaviors that prevented you from succeeding in your previous position. Split up from your spouse? Reduce the number of people and activities in your social life and concentrate exclusively on those that bring you joy.

How frequently you ought to do it

The benefit of going through a full life detox is that keeping your mind and spirit pure will be much simpler afterward. When the seasons change, plan maintenance weekends every three months and complete the task correctly the first time. It can greatly improve your quality of life and make it simpler for you to make wise decisions every day to regularly reflect on your life, get rid of things that no longer serve you, and add new and exciting things.

What you must first do

Primarily effort and time. Choose a week when you have a few other obligations and dedicate a few hours each night to your detox.

Supporting activities

Your body is supported while it works hard to rid itself of toxins by things like dry brushing, sauna sessions, yoga classes, and plenty of downtime. Your mind is the one that requires the most assistance during a life detox because purging your life can be mentally taxing.

Try the following daily, both before and after you cleanse a particular area of your life, for the best support for your mind and soul:

Pre-detox meditation and visualization

To meditate, take a few minutes to sit in silence. Imagine what it will be like to wake up to a tidy bedroom, how much fun it will be to cook in the decluttered kitchen, and how relieved it will make you to have a clean inbox and a well-organized phone. Consider the area of your life that needs detoxification today.

After-detox practice of self-kindness and gratitude

Make sure you intentionally disconnect from the mentally taxing work you just completed after your hard labor. Enjoy a cup of tea and a lovely, hot bath as a treat for yourself. Take a few minutes to sit in silence and pat yourself on the back for taking care of yourself.

Before you fall asleep, make sure you release any heavy emotions that your detox may have brought up. Make sure you get eight hours of rest.

Detox your habits

You are what you do every day, whether you like it or not. Our routines, customs, and habits make up our lives. Therefore, if you want a kickass existence, you need to have kickass habits.

Make a list of everything you do each week to help you detox your behaviors. Next, pose the following queries to yourself:

Will this habit help me achieve my goals? (Hint: binge-watching Netflix every night might not be the best way to achieve your side business objective.) Is this a habit I should get into? Do I love doing something, or am I just doing it out of habit or social pressure? (Hint: aimlessly perusing the internet late at night instead of going to sleep could negatively affect your quantity and quality of sleep). (Hint: just because you've been hanging out with your friends every Friday in the pub since you were in college doesn't imply you still love it.)

Less is definitely more in every other area (clothing, paperwork, emails), and you should clear the clutter before bringing new items into your life. But not with habits: generally speaking, it is much simpler to form new habits in place of old ones than it is to simply stop doing something. Choose a specific action you will perform in place of smoking whenever you feel the need (e.g., Take 5 deep breaths, take a stroll around the block) if your goal is to stop smoking.

Another way that habit-building differs from your other detoxing activities is that, instead of tackling everything at once and creating a clean slate, it is best to work on one habit at a time and move on to the next only after the first has truly become ingrained.

The O'Neill lifestyle

Well-known naturopath, author, and health educator Barbara O'Neill is well-known for her all-encompassing approach to wellbeing. In order to attain optimum health and fend against illness, she supports natural medicines and lifestyle modifications. The three main tenets of Barbara's philosophy are nutrition, detoxification, and the effectiveness of the body's natural healing processes.

Her teachings strongly emphasize the benefits of stress reduction, moderate exercise, whole-foods, plant-based diets, and proper water. She advocates staying away from refined sweets, processed meals, and dangerous chemicals. Rather, Barbara promotes the use of whole grains, organic fruits and vegetables, and natural supplements.

Barbara O'Neill also emphasizes the need to lead a well-balanced life that includes getting enough sleep, practicing mindfulness, and cultivating wholesome connections. Her techniques are based on contemporary scientific research and conventional wisdom, making her a well-respected authority in the natural health area.

By making educated, natural decisions, Barbara has motivated countless people to take control of their health through her books, seminars, and online tools. Her lifestyle advice is to complement the body's natural cycles and promote self-healing in order to empower people to live healthier, more energetic lives.

Daily routines for optimal health tips for sustainable living

Being the best version of yourself takes time, but we'll make it easier by providing you with some practical examples of healthy daily routines.

Drink a glass of lemon water to start the day

To enjoy a pleasant start to your day, simply squeeze half a lemon into your glass and sip.

Lemon juice lowers the acidity levels in your body, which helps shield you from inflammatory illnesses, including osteoporosis and fungal infections.

Workout in the early am

Exercise first thing in the morning enhances circulation, boosts energy, and promotes healthy lymphatic function. Every day, even only 20 or 30 minutes can have an impact! For overall health and toning, alternate between cardio and weight training during the week.

Another useful strategy for monitoring your weight is to go on the scale every morning. Weigh yourself every week; failing to do so will allow you to continue to deny that you have gained any weight.

Awesome breakfast

Make sure you fuel your body with a balanced meal that includes slow-release carbohydrates, protein, and vitamins and minerals. Low-sugar granola bars with a piece of fruit, veggie omelets, and yogurt with almonds and berries are all sensible choices.

Remain hydrated

It may surprise you to learn that even a small amount of dehydration can affect mood and focus. Water or other low-sugar beverages should always be available for consumption.

Eat a healthy lunch

Having a nutritious lunch may become a daily habit for even the busiest of us. You can prepare ahead of time and pack for work when it comes to lunch ideas.

Stay away from consuming too much fat at lunch because it will encourage afternoon sluggishness, which won't help you get through a busy day.

Do some mid-afternoon stretches

The majority of us experience a mid-afternoon "slump" between 2 and 4 pm, but you can avoid it by eating a nutritious lunch and engaging in some gentle exercise or stretches in the afternoon.

Dinner

It's never been easier to put a quick but healthful dinner on the table, thanks to the abundance of meal planning apps available! Make a practical choice that won't take much time or effort to put together. If not, you might order takeaway.

Due to their alkalizing properties and abundance of antioxidants, green veggies are always a fantastic option. Choose plant-based proteins like seitan or tofu to reduce acidity levels in the body. If you want animal protein, use lamb or fish instead of beef or chicken. [5]

Caffeine will keep you from getting a good night's sleep, so stay away from it in the late afternoon and evening.

Allow time to de-stress

While occasional stress is natural, prolonged periods of high stress put you at risk for depression and high blood pressure, among other illnesses and issues.

Choose a healthy hobby or pastime that helps you unwind, and then make time each day to include it in your schedule. This may be keeping a journal, reading a motivational book, petting a pet, practicing meditation, or just taking a moment to acknowledge all the positive things in your life.

Go to sleep at a reasonable hour

It should go without saying that getting enough sleep is essential for feeling your best. The majority of experts advise us to sleep between six and ten hours every night.

Avoid strenuous exercise in the late evening and turn off your computer and phone at least an hour before bed. When it comes time to go to bed, these steps will assist you in relaxing.

BOOK 8:

Rest and Emotional Wellness

Rest and rejuvenation

In the absence of a pandemic, Americans are under stress. Roughly one-third of respondents say they experience high stress, and up to three-quarters say stress negatively affects their mental health.

Better mental health, sharper focus and memory, a stronger immune system, less stress, happier moods, and even a faster metabolism all depend on getting enough sleep.

What do you mean when you say the term "rest"? When you are at rest, how do you imagine yourself spending your time?

We frequently underestimate the value of relaxation in today's fast-paced society, where hustle and production are praised. But did you know that getting enough rest is an essential part of a healthy lifestyle?

Let's first discuss more about the various forms of rest, as sleep is an essential part of rest and merits special attention. We'll explore the importance of rest in all its manifestations, highlight its amazing health benefits, and consider some practical ways to integrate this into our hectic schedules.

One definition of the term "rest" as a noun is a rejuvenating state of ease, quiet, or inactivity following an effort. Alternatively, resting means feeling refreshed or getting rid of fatigue.

That, in my opinion, has a lot to do with how frequently we consider the various forms of rest. Walking, yoga, meditation, and other forms of exercise are examples of activities that some of us may find to be conducive to active rest and renewal. However, some people may find that more passive rest involves less stimulating activities, such as napping or indulging in leisure pursuits like reading or listening to music.

Another way to classify rest is according to the aspects of our wellness that it replenishes:

Giving your body a vacation from physical activity and enabling it to heal is referred to as physical rest. This can be as simple as sitting, reclining, or lying down in a comfortable position. Physical rest aids in releasing tense muscles, lowering weariness, and encouraging general physical relaxation.

Giving your mind a vacation from constant mental stimulation and cognitive activity is known as mental rest. It's about giving your mind permission to unwind and rejuvenate. This can be accomplished by daydreaming, taking a break from work- related duties, or indulging in leisure pursuits or hobbies that don't require much mental concentration. Mental rest strengthens cognitive functioning, increases focus and creativity, and lessens mental tiredness.

Taking a vacation from emotional pressures and giving oneself time to emotionally recharge are both part of emotional rest. It's about finding ways to unwind and revitalize your emotions as well as making room for emotional well-being. Emotional rest can be attained by journaling, going outside, doing things that make you happy, or asking loved ones for emotional support. Emotional rest promotes emotional resilience, mood enhancement, and stress management.

In order to relieve sensory stimulation, sensory rest entails cutting back on or removing excessive sensory input. Sensory rest can be quite important in today's environment of bright lights, loud noises, and digital devices. It can be accomplished by turning off electronics, dimming lighting, spending time in a calm and quiet setting, or engaging in sensory-focused relaxation methods like progressive muscle relaxation or deep breathing. The nervous system is calmed, sensory overload is decreased, and a peaceful, well-being-promoting state is fostered through sensory rest.

We can all probably think of instances in our lives when we required those many forms of rest. However, were you able to identify it at that moment? Increasing our awareness of the requirements of our body and mind is essential to bringing about transformation. The next time you're feeling down, stressed, or having trouble focusing, I'd like you to consider these many types of rest. It could assist you in determining the best course of action to take in the little amount of time you have to obtain the most rest possible.

Ultimately, staying rested is essential to preserving our overall health and wellbeing. Rest helps to prevent injuries and enhance performance by giving our bodies time to heal. Additionally, it promotes a strong immune system, lessens inflammation, and helps with muscle recovery. Rest also decreases blood pressure and aids in stress management, both of which promote heart health. It is important to recognize the positive effects of rest on our mental and emotional health. Focus, concentration, and cognitive function can all be improved by taking regular breaks, practicing mindfulness, or just unplugging from electronics. Additionally, sleep aids in mood regulation, anxiety management, and stress reduction. It also facilitates the brain's ability to digest information, which develops creativity and problem-solving skills. You may be beginning to see by now how interrelated these various resting patterns are and how crucial it is to treat them all at once in order to attain total wellbeing. Incorporating a range of restorative activities that focus on rest—physical, mental, emotional, and sensory—can support optimal health and help preserve a good balance in our contemporary life.

The critical role of sleep

Sleep frequently suffers in a world that moves quickly and is overloaded with obligations, technology, and unending demands.

It is impossible to exaggerate the significance of sleep for our health, though.

Sleep is a complicated and essential physiological process that enhances general well- being; it is not just a condition of rest.

Sleep is essential for preserving and improving our health, from immune system support and physical restoration to cognitive performance and emotional stability. A basic biological function, sleep is essential for maintaining general health and wellbeing. The mission of sweet sleep studio is to raise awareness of the value of getting enough sleep and how it affects many different areas of our lives. The scientific data supporting the significance of sleep and its implications for optimal health will be discussed in this article.

The science of sleep: sleep is a complicated physiological state marked by distinct patterns of brainwave activity and a decrease in consciousness and sensory activity. Numerous studies have shown that sleep is crucial for maintaining memory, restoring cognitive function, and rejuvenating the body.

Cognitive restoration: the brain goes through important processes that improve and repair cognitive function when we sleep. Sleep helps learning and memory retention by allowing recently learned material to be consolidated. Furthermore, it enhances focus, attention, and problem-solving skills, enabling people to function at their best in a variety of cognitive tasks.

Memory consolidation: accompanying the movement of information from short- term to long-term memory, sleep is essential to memory consolidation. Memories are consolidated, reinforced, and incorporated into the body's already-existing knowledge base while you sleep. Enough sleep, both in terms of quantity and quality, is essential to maximizing this process and improving our memory recall.

Physical and immune system function: immune system and physical health are directly correlated with sleep. A higher chance of acquiring a number of chronic illnesses, including diabetes, obesity, and cardiovascular disorders, has been linked to inadequate sleep. Lack of sleep can also damage immunological function, increasing a person's susceptibility to illnesses and decreasing the body's capacity to successfully fight off diseases.

Emotional well-being and mental health: both emotional well-being and the best possible mental health depend on getting enough sleep. Anger, sadness, and other mood disorders can all be attributed to sleep deprivation. Chronic sleep issues have also been connected to a higher chance of mental health issues like mood disorders, anxiety disorders, and, in extreme situations, psychosis.

Techniques for relaxation and stress management

One excellent method for managing stress is to practice relaxation techniques. Relaxation is more than just having a hobby or finding mental tranquility. It's a procedure that mitigates the negative impacts of stress on your body and mind. Finding ways to unwind can help you manage the stress of daily life. Additionally, these solutions can help with chronic stress or stress associated with other health issues, including pain and heart disease.

Relaxation techniques can help you, regardless of how well-managed your stress is currently. It's simple to pick up basic relaxation techniques. Relaxation methods are low-risk and frequently cost nothing. Additionally, they are portable.

Start by finding easy ways to unwind so that you may begin to reduce stress in your life and enhance your general health and well-being.

Finding the best relaxation technique for you

After a demanding day, for a lot of us, unwinding is dozing off in front of the television on the couch. However, this has no effect in lessening the negative consequences of stress. Instead, you must initiate your body's natural relaxation reaction, a deeply resting condition that reduces stress, slows breathing and heart rate, lowers blood pressure, and rebalances the body and mind. This can be achieved through engaging in relaxation practices like yoga, tai chi, deep breathing, meditation, or rhythmic exercise.

For example, you can pay for a professional massage or acupuncture treatment, but most relaxation techniques can be done at home or with the help of an affordable smartphone app or free audio download. But it's crucial to keep in mind that not everyone responds well to the same relaxing methods. Each of us is unique. The approach that works best for you is the one that is able to focus your thoughts and trigger the relaxation response while also fitting into your lifestyle. This implies that figuring out the technique—or techniques—that works best for you may take some trial and error. Once you have, consistent practice can help you feel better physically and mentally, sleep better, experience less daily stress and worry, and enhance your general health and wellbeing.

Deep breathing

Focusing on deep, purifying breaths, deep breathing is an easy-to-use yet effective relaxing method. It offers a rapid method of reducing tension and is simple to learn and practice practically anywhere. Along with other calming components like aromatherapy and music, deep breathing is the foundation of many other relaxation techniques. You can get help during the process with applications and audio downloads, but all you really need is a few minutes and a peaceful area to sit or relax.

How to do deep breathing exercises

With your back straight, take a comfortable seat. Place a hand on your stomach and another on your chest.

Inhale using your nostrils. Raise the hand that is on your stomach. The hand resting on your chest should not move at all.

Squeeze out as much air as you can via your mouth while tensing your abdominal muscles. When you exhale, your other hand should move very little and the hand on your stomach should move in.

Breathe in via your nose and out of your mouth as usual. Try to breathe sufficiently to cause your belly to rise and fall. When you let go, count gently.

Try lying down if you have trouble breathing from your abdomen when seated. Place a little book on your tummy and take deep breaths such that the book rises and falls with each breath.

Progressive muscle relaxation

In a two-step procedure known as progressive muscle relaxation, various body muscle groups are systematically tensed and relaxed. Regular practice allows you to get intimately acquainted with the sensations of tension and total relaxation in various body areas. This might assist you in responding to the initial indications of the tense muscles that accompany stress. Your thoughts will unwind in tandem with your body.

For even more stress alleviation, try combining progressive muscle relaxation with deep breathing.

Using progressive muscular relaxation techniques.

If you have a history of back issues, muscular spasms, or other significant injuries that could be made worse by tensing your muscles, see your doctor first.

Attempt to tension only the muscles that are meant to be tense, starting at your feet and working your way up to your face.

Take off your shoes, undo your clothes, and settle in. Spend a few minutes taking calm, deep breaths in and out.

Turn your focus to your right foot when you're ready. Just take a time to notice the sensation.

Slowly stretch the muscles in your right foot as hard as you can. Hold for ten seconds. Let your foot relax. Pay attention to the tension leaving your body and the sensation of your foot going limp and relaxed.

Take a moment to remain in this calm state while taking slow, deep breaths.

Turn your focus to your left foot. Tension and release of muscles should be done in the same order.

Ascend gradually through your torso, tensing and relaxing the various muscular groups.

Try not to tighten any muscles other than those intended; this may require some effort at first.

Visualization

Visualization, also known as guided imagery, is a form of meditation in which you picture a peaceful setting in which you are free to release any tension and anxiety. Whether it's a serene woodland glen, a cherished childhood location, or a tropical beach, pick the environment that most soothes you.

By using an app or audio download to walk you through the images, you can practice visualization yourself or with assistance. Additionally, you can choose to perform your visualization in complete quiet or with the assistance of listening devices, such as calming music, a sound machine, or a recording that corresponds with the environment you've selected—for example, the sound of the waves breaking on a beach.

Mindfulness meditation

In recent years, mindfulness has gained immense popularity, resulting in media attention and support from prominent figures, corporate executives, and mental health professionals. What is mindfulness, then? With mindfulness, you may be totally present in the moment by shifting your attention from worrying about the past or the future to what is happening right now.

Yoga and tai chi

Deep breathing and a sequence of both moving and stationary positions are practiced in yoga. Yoga can help with anxiety, stress reduction, flexibility, strength, balance, and endurance. Yoga can cause injuries if it is performed improperly; therefore, the best way to learn is to take group courses, hire a private teacher, or at the very least, watch instructional videos. After you've mastered the fundamentals, you can practice by yourself or with other people, modifying your routine as necessary.

Tai chi

You've probably witnessed tai chi if you've ever seen a group of people in a park slowly moving in unison. Tai chi consists of a series of passive, flowing, gradual body movements. Your attention is kept in the present by concentrating on your breathing and movement, which helps you to relax and cleanse your mind.

Anticipate highs and lows. It may occasionally take some time and effort to begin experiencing the full benefits of relaxation techniques like meditation. The sooner you see results, the more persistent you should be. Don't give up if you miss a few days or even a few weeks. Simply start over and gradually gain your previous momentum.

Emotional and spiritual wellness

People have begun to pay greater attention to their spirituality and mental welfare throughout the last (nearly) year and a half. Wellbeing, self-care, and mental health have received a lot of attention. However, what is meant by spirituality? And what impact does that have on our mental and emotional well-being?

Understanding that there is something more than yourself and holding morals, values, principles, and beliefs that direct and give your life meaning are essential components of spiritual wellbeing. They also display your choices and activities.

Taking care of oneself is essential to emotional wellbeing. It's about unwinding, reducing tension, and loving and caring for oneself. It is about gaining inner power and self-assurance, which are frequently connected to your morals and spiritual well-being. Another aspect of emotional wellbeing is being aware of your constant learning and development.

While there are many different interpretations of spirituality, generally speaking, it entails the quest for purpose in life as well as a sense of connection to something more than ourselves. Many characterize spirituality as holy. Some claim it is a profound sensation of closeness and aliveness. It is critical to understand that each person's experience will vary.

The role of mind, spirit, and soul

Our physical bodies are typically the first thing that comes to mind when we think about health. We think about what we eat, how we exercise, how often we get checked out, and maybe even about our health issues. But being healthy extends beyond our bodily state. It is deeper and more all-encompassing. A condition of perfect balance between the body, mind, and spirit is called health. An individual's whole well-being is made up of this tripartite unity.

Understanding the harmony

In its purest form, health is more than just the absence of illness. It is our mental condition, our soulful involvement with life, and the dynamic and harmonious functioning of our bodily systems. It is about being mentally clear, spiritually calm, and physically fit. This perspective is also supported by the World Health Organization (WHO), which defines health as a condition of whole physical, mental, and social well-being rather than only the absence of illness or disability. This thorough explanation highlights the significance of holistic health, or the balance of the body, mind, and spirit.

Mind

There are stressors and sources of stress everywhere. We need to be aware of our own mental health and take action to safeguard or enhance it, whether it's due to a new project at work, a growing family, or the ever-increasing demands on our free time.

Achieving mental health may help us become more focused at work, fortify our love or social connections, broaden our perspective on life, and enhance our enjoyment of our free time spent with friends and family.

Several tactics to think about are:

Pay attention to the symptoms of stress. Speak with someone if you need help coping with life's stresses, and if necessary, seek professional assistance.

Take a break. Make time every day for yourself. Get away from the strains of life by reading a book, taking a stroll, meditating, enjoying a coffee, or listening to music. Make sleep your first priority. Sleep revitalizes our minds and facilitates clear, concentrated thinking. To make sure your mind gets the rest it needs, set a bedtime and stick to it.

Be willing to work on yourself. To develop your abilities and boost your confidence, consider taking an online course, finding a mentor, attending a workshop, or getting particular guidance.

Body

Everyone is aware of the best ways to take care of their bodies: eating healthier and exercising more. It's much easier said than done, though.

Here are some initial recommendations for taking care of your physical well-being and maintaining the "machine" that we all depend on yet occasionally overlook: The secret is to be moderate. Reduce the amount of bad food, alcohol, salt, and soft drinks (even those without added sugar!). Spend some time reading nutrition labels to identify better snack alternatives.

Make an effort to work out frequently. Look for methods to include physical exercise into your daily routine, such as going up stairs rather than using the elevator or participating with coworkers in a lunchtime organized sport. Choosing to stroll outside rather than have lunch at your desk will prove to be a significant advantage. Take the initiative. To stay on top of your health, make an appointment for routine dental and medical examinations. Consult your doctor about ways to enhance your physical health.

Focus on the fundamentals. Pay attention to your activity, hydration, food, and sleep. Set attainable objectives, acknowledge minor victories, and never give up!

Soul

There is more to spiritual wellness than religion or new age ideologies. Finding our purpose and direction in life, acknowledging our joys, and knowing how to be satisfied with our lot in life are all important steps toward improving our spiritual health.

The following advice can help you feel more spiritually well:

Be willing to socialize and engage in novel or challenging conversations with new individuals. Making connections with others exposes us to the viewpoints and experiences of others and helps us to be open to new ideas.

Change your surroundings. Go for a stroll outside, meet at a coffee shop, or request to work from home. Adding variation to your routine may boost motivation and enjoyment.

Give yourself to your desires. All activities that bring you joy and nourish your spirit should be prioritized in your life, such as creating art, baking, reading, going on nature hikes, camping, or doing manual labor.

Treat yourself with kindness. Give yourself permission to pause and not work continuously throughout the day. Allow your spirit to breathe and live in the present.

Mental and emotional well-being

Finding happiness might feel like a challenging endeavor at times. We all too easily lose sight of happiness, tranquility, and contentment. Emotional and mental health are more vital than ever during these trying times. These are the basis of a happy and healthy existence.

What is mental wellness?

A person is said to be in a state of mental wellness if they are able to work effectively and efficiently, recognize their own skills, and deal with life's typical stressors. It includes having an optimistic attitude on life, emotional resilience, and psychological stability. A sense of purpose, solid connections, a sense of happiness, and the capacity to manage stress successfully are all components of mental wellness, which goes beyond the absence of mental health issues.

What is emotional wellness?

The capacity to effectively manage life's stressors and adjust to change and challenging circumstances is known as emotional wellness. It entails being aware of our feelings, knowing how to communicate them constructively, and knowing when to ask for help when we need it. Self-care, stress reduction, relaxation, and the growth of inner strength are traits of emotional wellness. It all comes down to being aware of both good and bad emotions and being equipped with the knowledge and skills necessary to control and comprehend them. It also entails developing a great feeling of compassion and empathy for oneself and other people.

The interplay between mental and emotional health

While emotional health is centered on our capacity to properly regulate and express feelings, mental health largely relies on our cognitive processes and functioning. Mental and emotional health are closely related, even if they have different traits. Our emotions can influence our mental processes and vice versa. For example, thinking of bad ideas all the time might make you feel depressed or anxious. Similar to how strong emotions can impair our judgment, they can also affect how we make decisions. Both are vital to our general well-being, and they may both suffer greatly from an imbalance.

Why are mental and emotional well-being so important?

Mental and emotional health is essential for us to thrive and perform at our best in our everyday lives. They encourage:

Life satisfaction and mental and emotional well-being are inextricably intertwined. Physical health: mental and physical well-being are closely related to one another. For instance, chronic diseases like heart disease can be brought on by stress.

Relationships: our interactions with others are influenced by our mental and emotional states. Having a sound mental condition enables us to build wholesome connections.

BOOK 9:

Herbs for Common Chronic

Health Conditions

In today's fast-paced world, maintaining good health can be a challenge. Many people are turning to natural remedies to address common health issues, seeking holistic alternatives that have been used for centuries across various cultures.

Herbal remedies come in various forms, including teas, tinctures, capsules, and topical applications. Each method of use can offer different benefits, and the effectiveness can vary based on the form and preparation of the herb.

You can take proactive steps toward achieving and maintaining optimal health by incorporating herbal remedies into your daily routine. Whether you are dealing with minor ailments like headaches and colds or more persistent issues such as anxiety and high blood pressure, this guide aims to empower you with natural solutions that can complement your overall wellness journey.

This guide is designed to provide you with natural solutions to a wide range of health problems, focusing on the use of herbs and plant-based remedies.

Overcoming digestive disorders

Digestion issues arise for almost everyone occasionally. These are among the most frequent grievances raised in medical offices. However, gas, bloating, constipation, diarrhea, or heartburn are common symptoms for over 10 million people.

The digestive system is a complex and sensitive organ that is readily upset by various things.

How does the digestive system work?

Though it may appear that digestion just takes place in the stomach, it actually involves numerous organs and is a drawn-out process. They come together to form the digestive system.

When you chew, saliva in your mouth begins to break down the meal. This is where digestion starts. Food that has been chewed is transferred to the esophagus, a tube that runs from your throat to your stomach when you swallow. Food is forced down

your esophagus by muscular contractions to a valve at its base, which opens to allow food to pass into your stomach.

The stomach uses stomach acids to break down food. After that, the food enters the small intestine. Nutrients are absorbed there, where food is further broken down by the digestive secretions of various organs, including your gallbladder and pancreas. The remainder passes via your big intestine. Water is absorbed in the large intestine. The rectum and anus then carry the waste out of your body. Digestive issues can arise at any point along the journey.

Signs and symptoms of common digestive issues

Some of the most common symptoms include:

- Constipation

- Diarrhea

- Nausea

- Vomiting

- Indigestion/heartburn

- Bloating/gas

- Blood in stool

- Pain

- Difficulty swallowing

- Changes in appetite

- Weight loss

Ways to overcome digestive discomfort

The digestive system is a complex and sensitive organ that is readily upset by various things. Digestive problems are never enjoyable, but there are strategies to get over them:

Natural remedies

Ginger

All you need to alleviate mild intestinal discomfort is ginger. This popular treatment can help with indigestion, diarrhea, vomiting, upset stomach, and nausea. Ginger is widely available and comes in several forms. Try brewing ginger tea or incorporating ginger into your diet. Another effective remedy for an upset stomach is ginger ale but watch out not to drink too much of it since this might lead to another type of soreness. If you get stomach pain while out and about, ginger hard candies are a great and convenient solution.

Lemon-flavored water

Because of the strong acidity of lemons, adding fresh lemon juice to warm water might help ease digestive discomfort by breaking down any leftover food that may be upsetting the stomach. Add a squeeze of lemon to your ginger tea for even more relief.

Chamomile tea

Because of its anti-inflammatory qualities, chamomile tea is a great option for relieving upset stomach pain. Gas, bloating, irritable bowel syndrome, stomach cramps, and indigestion can all be relieved by chamomile.

Boost your consumption of fiber

For the digestive tract to remain healthy, fiber is essential. Increasing the amount of fiber in your diet can help reduce symptoms of digestive pain and may even be a long-term remedy. Ensuring that the digestive systems are functioning correctly, including fiber in your daily routine helps avoid future digestive discomfort and conditions, including diverticulosis, hemorrhoids, and irritable bowel syndrome.

The recommended daily fiber intake for men is 38 grams, while for women, it is 25 grams. However, the majority of adult Americans don't even get half of the daily recommended amount of fiber. It's simple to include natural sources of fiber in your diet. Some foods high in fiber include:

Fruits and vegetables include broccoli, artichokes, pears, strawberries, avocados, apples, bananas, and beets.

Grains and legumes, including quinoa, kidney beans, chickpeas, lentils, oats, and popcorn. Chia seeds, almonds, and even dark chocolate with 70% or more cacao content are excellent sources of fiber.

You might want to consider taking a daily fiber supplement if you still feel like you aren't getting enough fiber from whole foods. Many supplements have no taste and can be sprinkled directly into food or added to water.

Drink more water

Digestion problems might arise from dehydration, which is necessary for healthy digestion. One of the easiest ways to ease intestinal discomfort is to simply drink more water throughout the day. Try trading in drinks like soda, sports drinks, and coffee for water a few times a day. Additionally, attempt to have a large glass of water prior to eating. It will not only assist you in eating less, but it will also help your digestive tract get ready for the upcoming meal. While being hydrated is crucial to preventing upset stomachs, avoiding drinking water right before or right after a meal is best since it dilutes the stomach acid, which breaks down food.

Eight eight-ounce glasses of water should be consumed daily by the average person. Pay attention to your body; it can need more or less water depending on the situation to ease intestinal discomfort. The best action is to just sip water when you're thirsty.

Managing diabetes naturally

One of your main daily objectives when you have diabetes is to maintain your blood sugar levels within a healthy range. Effective strategies to reduce blood glucose include eating a diet high in nutrients, exercising regularly, and using drugs like metformin and insulin.

If you have diabetes, controlling your blood sugar is a lifelong endeavor. It aids in delaying or preventing diabetes-related problems, such as heart, kidney, eye, and nerve disorders, according to the centers for disease control and prevention (CDC). It has the power to completely alter the disease's path.

"People with type 2 diabetes should absolutely try to lower their blood sugar levels through dietary approaches first," says Jessica Crandall, Rd., CDCES, owner of Vital Rd., a Denver-based company that provides nutrition planning and health coaching. For certain individuals, it can aid in disease prevention and its actual reversal.

According to Crandall, occasionally, medicine can be completely avoided with a few significant lifestyle adjustments. It's not fun to poke yourself with insulin, she claims. "Because diabetes is a progressive illness, you really need to learn how to manage it."

Understanding the role of diet in diabetes

Did you know that controlling type 2 diabetes largely depends on diet? This chronic illness, which affects millions of individuals worldwide, arises when the body becomes resistant to the hormone insulin, which aids in blood sugar regulation.

Selecting the correct foods

A healthy diet can help control blood sugar levels and reduce the risk of diabetic complications such as nerve damage and heart disease. Make it a goal to eat a diet rich in nutrient-dense, low in sugar and refined carbohydrates. You can control your blood sugar levels by including a range of fruits, vegetables, whole grains, lean meats, and healthy fats.

Considering meal time and portion sizes

Meal timing and quantity should be considered in addition to choosing the right foods. Avoiding blood sugar peaks and troughs can be facilitated by eating smaller, more frequent meals spaced out throughout the day. Avoid skipping meals completely since this could cause blood sugar levels to drop dangerously low.

Staying hydrated

Maintaining hydration is just as important when managing type 2 diabetes, but only with meals. Drink lots of water to keep your body functioning properly and to remove excess sugar from your system.

Minor adjustments can have a significant impact

Though it may be challenging to alter your diet, it's important to remember that even small changes can have a big influence. For example, switching to water or unsweetened tea instead of sugary drinks may help you consume less sugar and improve your overall health. It may be helpful to speak with a licensed dietitian or diabetes educator to develop a customized meal plan that meets your unique needs. A proactive commitment to healthy nutrition is necessary for managing type 2 diabetes. Making full, nutrient-dense meal choices, paying attention to portion sizes and meal timing, drinking plenty of water, and making small dietary adjustments can all help you control your blood sugar and reduce your risk of developing diabetes- related complications.

Key herbs for blood sugar regulation

One term for diabetes is the "silent killer." When a person has diabetes, their body becomes less sensitive to insulin, which raises blood sugar levels. Being a chronic illness, one needs to rely on prescription medications for the rest of their life. And this can seriously impair one's financial situation. It's also not good for one's health. When taken over extended periods, the majority of these medications can be hazardous to other organs and have additional negative effects.

Alternative therapies are a great way to supplement diabetes medications. Alternative therapies such as naturopathy, acupuncture, and acupressure offer options for reducing reliance on pharmaceuticals. Numerous plants are used in naturopathy treatments to address hyperglycemia. The following herbs can help reduce blood sugar:

Rosemary

Rosemary is what gives soups and curries their wonderful scent. Rosemary not only helps with weight loss but also regulates blood sugar. Additionally, rosemary lowers low-density lipoprotein (LDL) and raises high-density lipoprotein (HDL).

Ginseng

Ginseng has long been used in oriental medicine for many centuries. It is anti-diabetic and possesses exceptional immune-boosting qualities. Ginseng slows down the body's rate of absorption of carbohydrates. Ginseng also quickens the pancreas's synthesis of insulin.

Sage

Studies have demonstrated that sage significantly lowers blood sugar levels, especially when taken without food. Sage improves diabetes management by secreting more insulin into the body. The best way to drink it is as tea.

Gymnemate sylvestre or gurmar

In India, ayurvedic treatments for diabetes have included this herb for ages. It contains gymnemic acids, which block the tongue's taste buds for sweet foods. This aids in the person's ability to curb sugar cravings—additionally, the herb aids in the blood's utilization of extra glucose.

Oregano

This herb treats high blood sugar in two ways. Suppressing appetite for sweets lowers blood sugar levels and stimulates the pancreas to produce more insulin. Some of the components in oregano help to mobilize glucose within the cells. In addition to strengthening immunity, it lowers the body's production of carbohydrates.

Aloe vera

In south America, Mexico, Australia, and India, the meaty plant is a vital component of complementary and alternative medicine. It cures dyspepsia and lowers bodily inflammation. Numerous chronic lifestyle diseases, including diabetes, are caused by inflammation within the body. Learn more about aloe vera's advantages for hair and skin.

Ginger

Indian and Chinese cuisines make heavy use of ginger. Diabetes has been treated using the pungent plant. It aids in boosting insulin secretion and makes the body more sensitive to insulin.

Fenugreek

Skin and stomach problems have been treated using fenugreek seeds and herbs. This herb also combats issues related to metabolism. Fenugreek fights diabetes and lowers blood glucose levels.

Incorporating exercise for diabetes management

Exercise is a crucial component of diabetes management, working in tandem with medicine and a healthy diet. The advantages of exercise cannot be overstated for those with diabetes and many other medical disorders. By lowering LDL and raising HDL, physical activity helps control weight, lower high blood pressure, and balance cholesterol levels. Additionally, it reduces stress, builds bone and muscle strength, and improves general wellbeing. Exercise provides the added benefits of lowering blood sugar and improving insulin sensitivity, which helps combat insulin resistance in people with diabetes.

See why it's so important to maintain an active lifestyle and get some practical advice on how to do so.

Exercises to help you manage type 2 diabetes

A varied range of activities should be incorporated into a well-rounded fitness regimen. Your strength, flexibility, and level of fitness can all be maintained and increased with these exercises. Here are some suggestions to get you going:

Walking

For many people, walking is a low-impact activity that they love. Increasing calorie intake can help lower cholesterol, blood pressure, and glucose. Additionally, walking briskly for 30 minutes—roughly 100 steps per minute—is a wonderful method to achieve the Ada's recommended daily allowance of cardiovascular activity.

You can also incorporate exercises like stair climbing into your walks to increase their intensity. However, if you had not been active prior to receiving your diabetes diagnosis, you might want to start out cautiously and work your way up.

Running

You can progress from brisk walking to running with the right instruction and your doctor's blessing. When engaging in this faster-paced activity, there is a lower chance of high blood pressure, high blood sugar, and high cholesterol.

Cycling

The popularity of stationary bikes has a purpose. Regular cycling can enhance your posture, balance, and heart and lung health, among other things. To begin with, though, you don't need to buy an expensive workout bike. You can try riding a stationary bike at your neighborhood gym or pick up an old bike and head outside. Additionally, studies indicate that cycling can help people with diabetes achieve better health outcomes.

Dancing

Workouts might be more enjoyable if you incorporate dance into your regimen. Dancing is a heart-healthy exercise that also raises blood sugar levels and improves fitness. According to one study, those with t2d who engaged in dance training were more driven to follow a schedule than those who engaged in other forms of physical activity.

Water aerobics

There are several justifications for doing your exercise in the pool. Swimming and other water exercises are easy on the joints and can lower blood sugar. T2d patients may also improve heart health, strength, and general fitness.

High intensity interval training

With HIIT, you alternate between extended periods of lower-intensity movements and brief bursts of high-intensity exercise. It can be added to a variety of exercises, such as cycling and jogging. HIIT may help lower your fasting blood sugar levels if you have type 2 diabetes.

Weight training

Weights and other equipment are used in this type of strength training to increase or preserve muscular mass and strength. Additionally, it might improve glucose tolerance and insulin sensitivity in t2d patients.

Yoga

Yoga combines breathing, meditation, and low-impact movement. It can enhance strength, flexibility, and balance. This is especially beneficial for older t2d patients who may be more likely to fall. You might be able to control your cholesterol and blood sugar levels with the practice.

Tai chi

Tai chi also incorporates breathing exercises, meditation, and low-impact movements. This age-old method enhances the range of motion, balance, and general health. Including it in your exercise regimen may also help to reduce blood sugar.

Pilates

Pilates is another low-impact workout option, and it belongs on this list for good reason. It strengthens your core and enhances your balance and posture with breathing exercises and repetitive motions. Additionally, a study found that pilates exercise improved blood glucose management in t2d individuals.

BOOK 10:

Heart Health and Respiratory Conditions

Heart health and hypertension

The risk of heart disease or stroke is greatly increased by high blood pressure or hypertension. This is a result of the artery lining being harmed by excessive blood pressure. As a result, plaque may accumulate and the arteries may narrow.

According to the centers for disease control and prevention (CDC), a person with hypertension is more likely to get a heart attack or stroke.

The arterial walls become damaged by high blood pressure. Damage to the arteries may increase their susceptibility to plaque accumulation, which may result in a blockage or decreased blood flow. A heart attack or stroke may result from the obstruction if it happens close to the heart or brain, respectively.

Seven out of ten individuals who have their first heart attack and eight out of ten who have their first stroke also have high blood pressure, according to the CDC.

Hypertension.

When a person's blood pressure is greater than usual, it can cause hypertension, also known as high blood pressure.

Blood pressure can fluctuate throughout the course of the day, but persistently high blood pressure can cause some health issues.

Systolic and diastolic blood pressure are two numbers that are involved. Less than 80 millimeters of mercury (mmhg) diastolic and less than 120 mmhg systolic is considered normal blood pressure.

The following measurements may point to high or raised blood pressure in an individual:

Elevated: a blood pressure reading between 120 and 129 mmhg at the systolic and less than 80 mmhg at the diastolic points.

A systolic blood pressure of 130–139 mmhg or a diastolic blood pressure of 80–89 mmhg is considered stage 1 hypertension.

A systolic blood pressure of 140 mmhg or higher, or a diastolic blood pressure of 90 mmhg or higher, is considered stage 2 hypertension.

According to the CDC, 47% of American adults suffer from high blood pressure, and just 1 in 4 of these individuals have their hypertension under control.

Heart conditions

The term "heart disease" covers a wide range of disorders that affect the heart. Heart disease comes in various forms, such as:

- Coronary artery disease

- Heart attack

- Heart failure

The most prevalent type of cardiac illness, according to the CDC, is coronary artery disease (cad). The heart's blood flow may be impacted by cad. A person may experience a heart attack if their heart does not receive enough blood.

About 659,000 trusted source Americans lose their lives to heart disease each year.

Stroke

A stroke happens when the arteries that supply the brain burst or get clogged. Brain cells and arteries may die if oxygen-rich blood is no longer flowing through the brain. Stroke is the top cause of disability and the fifth most common cause of death in the United States, according to the American heart association.

What are the symptoms of hypertension?

In most cases, hypertension is a quiet illness. Many will not show any symptoms at all. It could take years or even decades for the illness to worsen to the point where symptoms start to show. Even yet, other problems could be the cause of similar symptoms.

Severe hypertension symptoms can include:

- Flushing

- Blood spots in the eyes (subconjunctival hemorrhage)

- Dizziness

Contrary to common belief, nosebleeds and headaches are not usually associated with severe hypertension unless a person is experiencing a hypertensive crisis, according to the American heart association.

Taking frequent blood pressure readings is the most effective technique to determine whether you have hypertension. Most doctor's offices take a blood pressure reading every appointment.

Consult your doctor about your risks for hypertension and any additional readings you might require to help you manage your blood pressure if you only have annual physicals.

For instance, your doctor might advise getting your blood pressure checked twice a year if you have a family history of heart disease or other risk factors for the illness. This keeps you and your physician informed of any potential problems before they become serious.

Essential heart health nutrients and herbs

Dietary decisions can safeguard heart health. Foods like lentils, flaxseeds, green tea, and asparagus may be good for heart health. They offer fiber, vitamins, minerals, antioxidants, and other nutrients. You can take a lot of steps to maintain the health and absence of sickness in your heart.

You may limit the amount of stress in your life, exercise every day, stop smoking, and arrange an annual checkup.

Heart health can benefit from all of these factors. However, controlling your diet is one of the easiest lifestyle modifications that can improve your heart.

Approximately half of the approximately 6 million people who have heart failure will pass away within five years after receiving a diagnosis.

Eating meals heavy in fat, cholesterol, or sodium can be detrimental to one's heart health, according to the centers for disease control and prevention (CDC). Thus, nutrition is a smart place to start when trying to reduce your risk of heart disease.

Let's look at some of the greatest meals to maintain a strong and healthy heart.

Asparagus

Asparagus is a natural source of folate, which aids in the body's defense against the accumulation of homocysteine, an amino acid. Elevated homocysteine levels have been associated with a higher risk of heart-related disorders, including stroke and coronary artery disease.

Lentils, beans, peas, and chickpeas

Known as pulses or legumes, beans, peas, chickpeas, and lentils can all dramatically lower levels of low-density lipoprotein (LDL), or "bad cholesterol." they are also a great source of protein, fiber, and antioxidant polyphenols, all of which are good for your heart and overall health.

Berries

Antioxidant polyphenols found in berries can lower the risk of heart disease. Berries are low in fat and an excellent source of iron, calcium, fiber, folate, vitamin A, and vitamin C.

Broccoli

Certain tests have shown that steamed broccoli reduces cholesterol and prevents heart disease.

Flaxseed and chia seeds

As a plant-based source, alpha-linolenic acid and other omega-3 fatty acids are abundant in these seeds. Among the many positive benefits of omega-3s include their ability to reduce total cholesterol, LDL, and triglyceride levels. They also lessen the accumulation of fatty plaques in the arteries and lower blood pressure.

Omega-3 fatty acids reduce the risk of conditions like thrombosis and arrhythmias that can result in a heart attack.

Dark chocolate

Rarely does a food taste as well as it does healthfully (when consumed in moderation), like dark chocolate.

Scientists currently think that dark chocolate provides protection against atherosclerosis, a condition in which plaque accumulates inside the arteries, raising the risk of heart attack and stroke.

Two processes linked to atherosclerosis appear to be inhibited by dark chocolate: arterial stiffness and white blood cell adhesion, which is the process by which white blood cells adhere to blood vessel walls.

Moreover, research has shown that boosting the amount of flavanol in dark chocolate—the substance that gives it its flavor and appeal—does not lessen its health advantages.

Coffee

Coffee is another item that seems too good to be true. Regular coffee consumption was associated with a lower risk of heart failure and stroke, according to a recent study.

It is crucial to remember that this study, which evaluated Framingham heart study data using machine learning, can only detect correlations between variables; it is unable to definitively determine causes and effects.

Fish high in omega-3s

Fish is low in saturated fat but high in protein and heart-healthy omega-3 fatty acids. It is frequently advised that those who already have heart disease or are at risk of getting it should consume more fish to boost their intake of omega-3 fatty acids, which can reduce the risk of irregular heartbeats and slow the buildup of plaque in the arteries.

The American heart association (aha) recommends that we consume a 3.5-ounce portion of fatty fish, such as albacore tuna, salmon, mackerel, herring, lake trout, or sardines, at least twice a week.

Green tea

According to a 2011 systematic review, consuming green tea may help lower cholesterol, which is known to be a major risk factor for heart disease and stroke. However, the review could not determine the amount of green tea required for any health advantages.

An additional review examined the impact of green tea consumption on individuals with hypertension in 2014. According to the report, green tea can lower blood pressure. However, the investigators were unable to ascertain if this slight decrease could aid in the prevention of heart disease.

Nuts

Nuts that are good for the heart include almonds, hazelnuts, peanuts, pecans, pistachios, and walnuts. Protein, fiber, minerals, vitamins, and antioxidants abound in these nuts. Walnuts are a heart-healthy, on-the-go food that is rich in omega-3 fatty acids, much like flaxseeds and fish.

Liver

The liver is the organ meat with the highest nutritional content. Specifically, the abundance of folic acid, iron, chromium, copper, and zinc found in the liver contributes to blood hemoglobin levels and heart health.

Oats

Oatmeal may help lower the risk of heart disease because it is high in soluble fiber. Oat-based products dramatically lower LDL and total cholesterol without causing any negative side effects, according to a 2008 evaluation of the research.

Red wine

The antioxidants in red wine have been linked to several health advantages, according to numerous research. It seems unclear, nevertheless, that the advantages of antioxidants exceed the risks associated with alcohol consumption.

However, a recent study suggested that these same antioxidants might serve as the building blocks for a novel stent used in angioplasty procedures, which enlarge blocked or narrowed veins to treat atherosclerosis.

The same researchers are currently working on a new type of stent that distributes antioxidants similar to red wine into the bloodstream to aid in wound healing, stop blood clots, and lessen inflammation during angioplasty.

It is important to remember that consuming alcohol generally is bad for your heart. In actuality, consuming alcohol in moderation—if at all—is critically crucial for cardiovascular health.

Spinach

Regular use of high-quality magnesium sources can aid in the maintenance of a healthy cardiac rhythm. One of the healthiest foods to eat for magnesium is spinach, and eating popeye's favorite vegetable has a number of health advantages.

Tomatoes

Rich in nutrients, tomatoes may assist in maintaining the health of our hearts. The heart-healthy nutrients found in little red fruits include fiber, potassium, vitamin C, folate, and choline.

Potassium helps prevent kidney stones from developing, strengthens muscles and bones, and staves against heart disease.

Researchers have shown that the most significant dietary modification to lower the risk of heart disease is to increase potassium intake while reducing sodium intake.

Veggies

According to the aha, eight or more portions of fruit and vegetables should be consumed each day. Vegetables are high in fiber, vitamins, and minerals but low in fat and calories. Blood pressure and weight can be moderated with a diet rich in vegetables.

Herbs and spices for heart health

Some people resort to natural therapies to maintain their hearts' health. Many populations have employed herbs and spices to treat their ailments for thousands of years. Try flavoring your food with these delectable herbs and spices to help improve heart health.

Certain pharmaceuticals and natural cures may not work well together. Using these herbs to season food is usually safe. But before including them in your diet, it's crucial to conduct thorough research and see your doctor if you're considering taking them as supplements.

What's the difference between herbs and spices?

Although they are both derived from plants, herbs and spices are comparable. Still, herbs are usually made from fresh plant material. Spices are typically derived from the dry, underground portion of plants. Herbs and spices both offer health advantages and can be used to enhance food flavor.

Try these heart-healthy herbs and spices:

Cinnamon.

Delicious cinnamon is a terrific addition to your favorite breakfast and dessert recipes. Its pleasant scent makes it popular throughout the winter holidays.

For thousands of years, people have used cinnamon, which is cherished for its many therapeutic benefits. Its capability to reduce harmful cholesterol levels is one such quality. It may also cause your blood pressure to drop. According to studies, a daily sprinkle of cinnamon may even help lower your risk of heart disease.

Garlic

Although it smells strongly, garlic can enhance the flavor of your foods. It also improves the health of your heart. This everyday kitchen item may provide relief from a number of ailments, including infections, high blood pressure, and the common cold.

Reduced blood pressure, bad cholesterol, and edema can all be achieved with fresh garlic. Garlic may lower your risk of heart attack or stroke in this way.

Cayenne

You're in luck if you enjoy a little spicy spice added to your dish. Cayenne pepper facilitates healthy blood circulation throughout the body. One of the compounds in cayenne that may help decrease blood pressure is called capsaicin. A healthier heart is one that has greater blood flow and less blood pressure.

Turmeric

The vibrant yellow spice turmeric is a mainstay in Indian cuisine. Even if you haven't experimented with this kind of cooking, you've undoubtedly heard about turmeric's health advantages. Turmeric gets its yellow hue from curcumin. It's also the source of the spice's health advantages.

Curcumin may have anti-inflammatory, anti-bad-cholesterol, and anti-blood-clot properties. Research also supports the health benefits of turmeric, which many people swear by.

Ginger

Tea, baked goods, Asian cuisine, and salads all benefit greatly from the inclusion of ginger. Studies reveal that consuming ginger daily can also help lower blood pressure, lower cholesterol, and maintain elastic and open blood vessels. According to studies, consuming ginger prevents those arteries from hardening, which suggests that it may be a useful herb for treating and preventing cardiac problems.

Coriander

Worldwide, coriander is an herb that is utilized in cuisine. Additionally, populations with high coriander consumption also have some of the lowest incidences of heart disease.

Never knew what coriander was? It's more often referred to as cilantro in the us. Despite their differences, these two are derived from the same plant.

This herb may assist in decreasing blood pressure and bad cholesterol, two risk factors for heart disease. Coriander can lower blood pressure because it acts as a diuretic, which is a chemical that removes excess fluid and sodium from the body.

Diet and lifestyle for blood pressure management

One billion individuals globally and about half of adult Americans suffer from high blood pressure. High blood pressure increases the risk of heart disease and stroke if it is not managed. Still, you can follow several natural methods in addition to taking medicine to help lower your blood pressure.

In order to effectively cure high blood pressure, lifestyle is crucial. Maintaining a healthy lifestyle and controlling blood pressure can help avoid, postpone, or minimize the need for medication.

These lifestyle modifications can effectively reduce and maintain low blood pressure.

Watch your waist size and shed those excess pounds

Weight gain is commonly associated with elevated blood pressure. Additionally, being overweight can lead to sleep apnea, which is a disorder of breathing during sleep that elevates blood pressure even more.

One of the best lifestyle adjustments for lowering blood pressure is losing weight. Even a modest weight loss can help lower blood pressure if you are obese or overweight. Blood pressure may generally decrease by around 1 millimeter of mercury (mm hg) for every kilogram (2.2 pounds) of weight loss.

Additionally, the waistline's size matters. High blood pressure risk might be increased by obesity around the waist.

Generally speaking, males with a waist measurement over 40 inches (102 cm) are in danger.

If a woman's waist measures more than 35 inches (89 cm), she may be at risk. Different ethnic groups have different numbers. Ask your healthcare professional to find out what a healthy waist measurement is for you.

Engage in regular exercise

Regular exercise can lower approximately 5 to 8 mm hg from high blood pressure. In order to prevent blood pressure from rising again, it's critical to continue exercising. Aim for at least 30 minutes of moderate physical activity daily as a general objective.

Additionally, exercise helps prevent high blood pressure, or hypertension, from developing from higher blood pressure. Frequent exercise helps lower blood pressure in hypertensive individuals to safer levels.

Aerobic exercises such as walking, jogging, cycling, swimming, or dancing can help reduce blood pressure. High-intensity interval training is another option. Short bursts of vigorous exercise are interspersed with slower intervals of activity during this kind of training.

Additionally, strength exercise helps lower blood pressure. Make an effort to work out with strength training at least twice a week. Consult a medical professional about creating an exercise regimen.

Consume a balanced diet

Up to 11 mm hg can be taken off of high blood pressure by eating a diet high in whole grains, fruits, vegetables, low-fat dairy products, and low in cholesterol and saturated fat. Dietary approaches to stop hypertension (dash) and Mediterranean diets are two examples of diets that can lower blood pressure.

Dietary potassium helps mitigate the blood pressure-raising effects of salt (sodium). Foods like fruits and vegetables are the finest sources of potassium, not supplements. Aim for 3,500–5,000 mg daily since this may result in a 4–5 mm hg drop in blood pressure. Find out how much potassium you should consume from your healthcare provider.

Cut back on sodium, or salt, in your diet

Reducing sodium consumption even slightly can positively impact heart health and lower high blood pressure by 5 to 6 mm hg.

The impact of salt consumption on blood pressure differs amongst demographic groups. Generally speaking, keep your daily sodium intake to 2,300 mg or fewer. For most adults, though, a daily consumption of 1,500 mg or less of salt is recommended. To cut back on salt consumption:

Examine the labels on food. Seek for foods and beverages that have reduced salt content.

Reduce your intake of processed foods. Foods only contain trace amounts of sodium by nature. Processing adds the majority of the sodium.

Leave out the salt. Use spices or herbs to give food flavor. Cook. You can regulate the food's salt content by cooking it.

Limit your alcohol intake

Reducing alcohol consumption to no more than one drink for women or two for men each day will help reduce blood pressure by roughly 4 mm hg. Twelve ounces of beer, five ounces of wine, or 1.5 ounces of 80-proof liquor make up one drink.

However, excessive alcohol use can cause blood pressure to rise several points. Additionally, it may lessen the benefits of blood pressure drugs.

Give up smoking

Blood pressure rises during smoking. Giving up smoking reduces blood pressure. Additionally, it can enhance general health and lower the risk of heart disease, which may prolong life.

Get a good night's sleep

Less than six hours of sleep per night for a few weeks is considered poor sleep quality and can lead to hypertension. Many conditions, such as sleep apnea, restless legs syndrome, and insomnia in general, can interfere with sleep.

If you frequently have problems falling asleep, let your healthcare professional know. Sleep can be improved by identifying the cause and addressing it. But if you don't suffer from rls or sleep apnea, try these easy sleep hacks for a more peaceful night's sleep.

Maintain a sleep routine. Set a daily routine for when you go to bed and wake up. Attempt to maintain a consistent routine on weeknights and weekends.

Make a peaceful environment. This calls for maintaining a cool, peaceful, and dark sleeping area. Spend the hour before going to bed doing something calming. This could be practicing relaxation techniques or having a warm bath. Steer clear of bright light sources like computer or tv screens.

Keep an eye on what you eat and drink. Avoid going to bed full or hungry. Aim to avoid heavy meals right before bed. In addition, limit or stay away from alcohol, caffeine, and nicotine right before bed.

Limit your naps. Resting naps during the day to no more than 30 minutes may improve evening sleep for people who find naps during the day beneficial.

Reduce stress

Chronic (long-lasting) emotional stress may be a factor in elevated blood pressure. More research is required to determine whether stress-reduction methods can lower blood pressure.

Finding strategies to lessen stress and identifying the sources of stress—such as job, family, money, or illness—can't hurt, either. Try this out:

Don't try to take on too much. Prioritize your tasks and make a plan for the day. Acquire the ability to refuse. Give yourself adequate time to complete the tasks at hand.

Make strategies to address the problems you can manage and concentrate on them. Speak to a supervisor about a problem at work. Look for solutions to resolve conflicts with your spouse or children. Steer clear of stressful situations. For instance, travel at a different time or use public transit if rush-hour traffic stresses you out. If at all possible, stay away from stressful people.

Set some time to unwind. Every day, set aside some time to sit still and really breathe. Allocate time for pleasurable pursuits or interests, including hiking, cooking, or volunteering.

Show appreciation for what you have. Giving thanks to other people helps ease tension.

Keep an eye on your blood pressure at home and schedule regular checkups

You can monitor your blood pressure at home with the aid of monitors. It can confirm that the adjustments in your lifestyle and drugs are effective.

There are many readily available, non-prescription home blood pressure monitors. Before you begin, discuss home monitoring with a medical professional.

Another essential component of blood pressure management is routine provider visits. Find out from your doctor how frequently you should get your blood pressure checked if it is under control. It may only be possible for you to examine it once a day or less frequently.

Natural solutions for respiratory conditions

Respiratory ailments such as emphysema, asthma, or chronic obstructive pulmonary disease (COPD) can have a serious negative effect on your loved ones' quality of life. These days, natural therapies may be found everywhere. Everyone is promoting their own version of a remedy for whatever ails you, from zinc to vitamin C. And the conversation certainly gets heated during the fall and winter respiratory sickness season.

Herbal remedies for asthma and allergies

Certain foods and herbs can help reduce inflammation, fight oxidative stress, and strengthen the immune system, all of which can help reduce asthma symptoms. These consist of garlic, ginseng, and turmeric.

Can herbs help with symptoms of asthma?

For those who suffer from asthma, immune-boosting herbs can be especially helpful because a robust immune system can better handle triggers and potentially lessen the frequency of asthma attacks. Antioxidants may aid in the management of asthma because oxidative stress in the lungs can cause inflammation and restriction of the airways.

The inflammation associated with asthma causes the airways to swell and narrow, resulting in symptoms such as coughing, chest tightness, wheezing, and shortness of breath. Certain herbs have the potential to mitigate these symptoms by decreasing inflammation.

Herbs remedies for asthma

Turmeric

This vibrant yellow spice is probably already in your cabinet, where it may be used to make curries and other tasty foods. Curcumin is what gives turmeric its color. Additionally, this natural coloring ingredient has anti-inflammatory properties.

Both cancer and arthritis may benefit from turmeric. One trial on asthma included 77 people with mild to moderate asthma who took curcumin pills for a duration of 30 days.

Researchers discovered that the supplement lessened blockage of the airways and may be a useful adjunctive asthma treatment. Keep in mind that this is just one tiny study; additional research is required to ascertain the advantages and disadvantages.

Garlic and ginseng

Common herbs like ginseng and garlic can be found in a range of supplement formulations.

Some suggest that ginseng, an Asian plant, has numerous health advantages, including treating respiratory ailments. Significant health advantages, including lowered blood pressure and cholesterol, are also believed to come from garlic.

A tiny study on rats found that taking ginseng and garlic supplements helped lessen asthma symptoms.

Rats were subjected to an agent that affected the lungs during the trial. During the exposure, the researchers gave the rats ginseng and garlic. Compared to the other group, those who received the herbs had a reduction in symptoms and inflammation. However, additional human research is required to validate the efficacy of these botanicals.

Chinese herb mixtures

Researchers have examined the efficacy of herbal remedies from traditional Chinese medicine for asthma over the past few decades.

Among them is the combination known as anti-asthma herbal medication intervention (ASHMI). This mixture contains ku shen (sophora root), gan cao (licorice root), and lingzhi (a fungus). Some say that, in contrast to steroid drugs, this combination of herbs can lower inflammation and constriction of the airways while maintaining elevated cortisol levels.

The efficiency of ASHMI has been the subject of several investigations. A study conducted on mice found that the herbal mixture reduced the symptoms of asthma. In a different trial, researchers examined the efficacy of ASHMI in 20 asthmatic non- smokers. They discovered that individuals had good herbal tolerance and that ASHMI seemed to be safe.

Other Chinese herb combinations, including modified mai men dong tang, may be useful in treating asthma. This herbal mixture was found to alleviate symptoms of mild-to-moderate asthma in 100 individuals without causing any negative effects. Throughout the trial, all individuals combined the use of botanicals with conventional western asthma treatments.

However, there is a dearth of research because most of these studies are conducted on animals or with small numbers of individuals.

Black seed

Nigella sativa is another name for this spice. According to certain research, it may have therapeutic advantages, such as easing the symptoms of asthma.

In order to evaluate the efficacy of black seed and asthma, one researcher looked at earlier studies. The study came to the conclusion that other studies have suggested black seed may benefit airway function, inflammation, and asthma symptoms. It also highlighted how much more research is required.

Honey

This natural and delicious material might help with several parts of your asthma. Honey has the ability to soothe your respiratory tract and lessen the tickling that makes you cough. Adults who are coughing less at night can take two teaspoons of honey.

You can even infuse honey with medicines like turmeric to further reduce your symptoms.

In rabbits with asthma, honey has been demonstrated to alleviate symptoms. In one study, 40 rabbits with asthma had fewer symptoms after receiving honey that had been turned into a gas.

However, this does not imply that honey can lessen a person's symptoms of asthma. More research is required to find out if this honey dispensing technique can benefit those who have asthma.

Herbs that help to fight respiratory allergies

Many persons in all age groups are vulnerable to respiratory allergies or the exacerbation of preexisting conditions due to the pollution levels' refusal to drop to a safer range. It's crucial to exercise extra caution if you have a respiratory illness like asthma, bronchitis, or allergies, particularly when the weather or season changes.

Herbs for alleviating respiratory allergies:

While it's crucial to take prescription drugs exactly as directed by a physician, those who occasionally experience respiratory issues may find relief by using certain natural herbs in their daily routine. These natural herbs will aid in the treatment of typical respiratory allergy symptoms.

Eucalyptus oil

Although eucalyptus is thought to be native to Australia, it is a popular herb throughout the Indian subcontinent. Its distinct scent sets it apart from the other essential oils and helps it work as a natural therapy for a variety of ailments, including allergies related to the respiratory system. The oil's remarkable medical qualities can be attributed to its abundance of anti-inflammatory and antibacterial characteristics. This oil soothes and treats respiratory and nasal allergies. By acting on the sinus and nasal passages, it lessens inflammation.

Oregano

The majority of us are familiar with using oregano as a garnish for soups, pasta dishes, and pizzas. But this flavorful, widely used culinary herb also has a wealth of therapeutic uses. Yes, oregano naturally has anti-allergic and decongestant properties. This explains why respiratory allergies are frequently treated with this plant.

Peppermint oil

This is the solution if you've been coughing, sneezing, and having eye irritation all day. Leaves of peppermint have a calming effect on the skin and throat. This is because it includes menthol, which has the dual effects of calming the respiratory tract and relaxing the muscles of the respiratory tract. In addition to being a decongestant and antihistamine, peppermint is a fantastic herbal medicine for persons with inflammation, allergies, coughing, and sore throats.

Nettle leaf

The advantages of nettle leaf are not widely known. It functions as a naturally occurring antihistamine, meaning that it stops your body from making histamine, which is what triggers allergic reactions. This leaf has strong analgesic, antibacterial, and anti-inflammatory qualities and is sold at ayurvedic stores.

Chamomile oil

This one is one of the most well-liked and effective herbs for respiratory issues. It possesses amazing antispasmodic, antihistamine, anti-inflammatory, and antioxidant qualities. This implies that it will combat the majority of allergy symptoms, such as irritation, inflammation, and itching. Therefore, it is advisable to get chamomile oil if you have any respiratory issues because it has a general benefit and few negative effects.

BOOK 11:

Skin Conditions and Mental Health

Addressing skin conditions with herbs

Since ancient times, herbal treatments have been used to cure a wide range of conditions, from cancer to minor stomach upsets. The use of herbs in the treatment of a variety of medical conditions is supported by recent research.

But a lot of people who think that "natural" is preferable have attempted untested, unregulated remedies, sometimes with unsatisfactory or even harmful outcomes. Certain common skin diseases can be effectively treated with herbal remedies; visiting the doctor is not always necessary.

Dr. Doris Day, a clinical assistant professor of dermatology at NYU medical center and a dermatologist in Manhattan, suggests that "Aloe vera is the best herbal cure for treating skin issues if I could only use one. It is well known that this plant has unique therapeutic properties." Pure aloe vera is used as a moisturizer and skin softener. For generations, people have utilized the gel, or the liquid found inside the leaves, to hasten the healing of wounds. It acts as a topical pain relief in addition to promoting healing. Dr. Day continues, "Unfortunately, a large number of aloe vera-containing products in stores do not contain enough of the ingredient to be helpful." Aloe vera is a very efficient treatment for psoriasis. This very common disorder causes itchy, red, scaly areas on the skin and scalp, according to several credible studies.

Arnica flower formulations applied topically are very beneficial for wound healing. It works well as an antibacterial, anti-inflammatory, and analgesic (pain reliever). "This treatment is indicated for bruises and swelling related to trauma or surgery," says Dr. Day in his additional remarks. Additionally, it relieves joint discomfort and accelerates the healing of minor skin abrasions and bug bites. Arnica has been authorized by the German government to be used as a wound-healing remedy.

Calendula flower, also referred to as common marigold, has a long history of being used to treat cuts, rashes, burns, bruises, and skin diseases. Its application as a topical treatment for wounds that are not healing well, as well as for specific kinds of skin ulcers, has been approved by the German health authorities. Calendula tea compresses are also beneficial. Tea can be used as a mouthwash to treat painful oral sores.

For generations, people have utilized comfrey's leaves and roots to speed up the healing of injuries and bruises. It's proved helpful in treating rashes as an anti- inflammatory as well. When applied to the skin over the injury site, it is believed to accelerate the healing of closed fractures. While using the roots or leaves topically is harmless, dr. Day cautions against applying them over broken skin since this can cause toxicity and should not be done more than three days in a row. Comfrey leaf tea has additional benefits, but you shouldn't drink more than three cups a day.

Tall evergreen tea trees can be found in Asia and Australia. The leaves were used as a disinfectant during World War I and as an antiseptic for millennia. Insect bites, wounds, and other common skin issues have been treated using leaf oil in more recent times. It has been demonstrated that the oil kills bacteria and fungi. The oil is sold in stores without a prescription and can be diluted to suit different medical needs. It is never advisable to use tea tree oil orally due to potential toxicity.

For thousands of years, chamomile has been used to treat a wide range of medical issues. Tea produced from dried and fresh flowers has been used topically to promote wound healing and cure moderate skin conditions like sunburn, rashes, and itchy lesions. It has also been used as an oral rinse to treat gingivitis and unpleasant mouth sores.

Known by many as cayenne, this hot red pepper has been used as a remedy for a wide range of illnesses, including high blood pressure, ulcers in the stomach, poor circulation, lung infections, and skin infections. Capsaicin is often combined with other herbal items in formulae to enhance its antibacterial and anti-inflammatory properties. Dr. Day claims that capsaicin is a potent analgesic because it has been demonstrated to remove substance-p from nerve endings. Due to the release of substance-p, there may initially be a burning feeling or an increase in pain. These effects are often transient.

Numerous herbal treatments are effective in treating common skin disorders. According to Dr. Day, if a person taking some herbal medicines is susceptible to any of the active substances, they may experience negative side effects. If your skin condition doesn't go away or your symptoms worsen, you should visit your doctor.

Herbal treatments for acne, eczema, and psoriasis

Long-term skin illness and acne are brought on by clogged hair follicles, oil from the skin, and dead skin cells. Up to 85% of youths in North America are impacted. The skin regions most commonly affected by acne are the face, upper chest, and back because they have a comparatively high concentration of oil glands. Pimples, greasy skin, blackheads or whiteheads, and maybe scarring can all be signs of acne-prone skin. Combining Chinese medicinal herbs, facials, and dietary changes can be used to treat acne.

Best herbs for acne

It's important to comprehend the physiology of the skin and how herbal medicines might assist its well-being before getting into specific plants. Excess sebum, dead skin cells, and bacteria that cause acne block pores, causing inflammation and the development of pimples, blackheads, and whiteheads. You may naturally address these core issues by including the appropriate herbs in your skincare routine.

Witch hazel: the astringent that tightens pores

Because of its astringent properties, witch hazel is well known for its ability to tighten and tone pores. This herb soothes sensitive skin and lowers sebum production, which helps to reduce inflammation and the appearance of acne breakouts.

Including witch hazel in your daily direct application routine: after cleansing, use a witch hazel toner to tighten pores and get the skin ready for moisturizer.

Spot treatment: to calm the skin and lessen redness, apply a cotton ball immediately to the irritated area.

The antiseptic warrior: tea tree

With its exceptional antibacterial and anti-inflammatory qualities, tea tree oil has long been a mainstay in the treatment of acne. This powerful oil, which is derived from melaleuca alternifolia plants, works to treat acne by deeply infiltrating pores, cleaning them, and destroying bacteria that cause acne.

Techniques for applying tea tree directly on acne: using a cotton ball, dab tea tree oil onto imperfections after diluting it with a carrier oil.

Add a few drops to your usual cleanser to increase its antibacterial properties. Diy masks: add it to clay masks to improve the pore-cleansing action.

Neem: the antimicrobial superhero

An excellent treatment for acne, neem is an herb with a long history in ayurvedic medicine. It is known for its antibacterial and anti-inflammatory qualities. Neem leaves and oil are used to treat a variety of skin issues, including severe acne.

Techniques for applying neem oil: to reduce inflammation and fight infection, apply diluted neem oil to the affected regions.

Neem leaf paste: for a more thorough treatment, make a paste out of crushed leaves and use it as a face mask.

Aloe vera: the calming agent

The well-known herb aloe vera soothes irritated skin and hydrates without blocking pores. Anti-inflammatory qualities found in aloe vera gel aid in treating and reducing acne lesions.

How to use aloe vera gel effectively: apply fresh aloe vera gel straight to the skin as a soothing gel for irritated regions or as a moisturizer.

Added to lotions: combine aloe vera gel with your regular moisturizer for more hydration and therapeutic effects.

The anti-inflammatory soother: chamomile

In addition to having relaxing properties when drunk as a tea, chamomile has antibacterial and anti-inflammatory properties that aid the skin. For delicate skin that could respond negatively to heavier topical acne treatments, it's a great option.

Uses of chamomile for acne

Toner for chamomile tea: apply chilled chamomile tea as a mild skin toner to reduce redness and swelling.

Oil infused with chamomile: use chamomile-infused oils to calm and repair the skin around acne lesions.

Herbs high in salicylic acid: the natural exfoliants

Salicylic acid is a beta-hydroxy acid that is well-known for its capacity to unclog pores and exfoliate skin. Although it is frequently present in over-the-counter acne treatments, this component occurs naturally in some herbs, providing a gentler pore cleaning and exfoliating method.

Applications of salicylic acid-rich herbs

Extract from willow bark: apply lotions that include salicylic acid from willow bark extract, a natural source, on your skin to gently exfoliate and soothe inflammation. Extracts from berries: strawberries, in particular, have a natural salicylic acid content. Make your own masks with berry extracts for a mild exfoliation treatment.

Herbs for eczema & psoriasis

Psoriasis and eczema are examples of skin disorders that can be annoying. They are infamously hard to treat and result in red, itchy spots on the skin. Topical anti- inflammatory creams are the standard treatment for these disorders; however, they typically only offer momentary or limited respite. Recurrence occurs often.

This therapy approach has an issue because it targets the symptom (branch) of the illness rather than the underlying cause (root). The approach used in traditional Chinese medicine is different. We investigate beneath the surface to identify the condition's underlying cause, which may surprise you. When utilized properly, herbs can treat the underlying causes of these annoying disorders in addition to their symptoms, providing a unique option for treating them. These are my top six favorite herbs for psoriasis and eczema.

Turmeric (curcuma longa) is one of the most well-known plants in the world. It is a golden root. It has been used for hundreds of years, yet people still use it today as a superfood and herbal remedy. Turmeric has several health benefits, but its anti-inflammatory and antioxidant properties are the plant's two most powerful attributes.

Turmeric has an effect on almost every organ in the body. It soothes the skin, lessens intestinal tract inflammation, and enhances liver detoxification.

Poor hepatic or intestinal clearance is the cause of most occurrences of psoriasis and eczema. These organs are responsible for safely removing harmful waste products from the body.

Polypodium leucotomos, or samambaia

Samambaia, a lowly fern native to south America, follows turmeric's rise to fame. Outside of Brazil, samambaia has been able to stay out of the spotlight for a long time.

It works specifically for skin disorders, including psoriasis and eczema and also strengthens the skin's defenses against UV radiation from the sun. It functions by stopping the inflammatory mechanism that causes these ailments.

More precisely, samambaia is a strong inhibitor of nuclear-factor kappa b, an important inflammatory sign. This is the main indicator of inflammation linked to psoriasis and a moderating factor in eczema.

Sillybum marianum, or milk thistle

When it comes to supporting liver function, milk thistle is among the greatest herbs available. It is known as a "hepatoprotective" among herbalists. Since the Latin word hepato means "liver," milk thistle is primarily referred to as a "liver defender."

In fact, milk thistle is the sole recognized treatment for several liver poisonings found in the world of plants and fungi.

By strengthening the liver cells' capacity to eliminate substances from circulation, milk thistle significantly enhances liver function and relieves skin tension. The faster our skin returns to normal, the more efficiently toxins are handled by the liver, as they should.

Calendula: topical (calendula officinalis)

Calendula is an herb that many herbalists recommend when asked about their preferred herb for irritation of the skin.

This little flower may seem innocent, but its petals are powerful. Tnf-alpha is one of the main inflammatory markers that they block, along with cox and 5 lox, two of the main enzymes that cause inflammation. These pro-inflammatory chemicals are important in the development of eczema and psoriasis.

Aspirin, a popular anti-inflammatory medication, also targets one of these enzymes, called cox.

Calendula has immediate anti-inflammatory, nourishing, and vulnerary (promotes healing) properties when applied topically to the skin.

Because it supports the symptoms and speeds up skin healing, this herb works well when combined with some of the other herbs on our list. It is less effective, though, at curing the underlying cause of many ailments.

Sarsaparilla (smilax spp.)

Nearly every continent is home to several species of sarsaparilla plants. Sarsaparilla has been utilized as a skin and liver disease remedy by almost all indigenous cultures that inhabit the places where it grows.

Sarsaparilla is used in traditional Chinese medicine to remove "blood heat," which is considered to be one of the main causes of psoriasis.

Sarsaparilla purges the blood by binding and eliminating a large number of harmful substances that are in the bloodstream. Sarsaparilla also improves digestive function and liver detoxification, which addresses the underlying causes of psoriasis and eczema.

German chamomile: topical (matricaria recutita)

Most people know that chamomile tea works well as a natural sleep aid and stress reliever. Most people are unaware that chamomile has specific advantages for the skin and is also a strong pain reliever and anti-inflammatory.

A topical use of diluted essential oil, such as olive or coconut oil, can be used to soothe skin issues. Even better, think about diluting a calendula oil preparation with a few drops of chamomile essential oil.

German chamomile is more effective in alleviating the symptoms, much like calendula. Specifically, skin irritation. It is an excellent treatment for severe itching and tingling due to its anti-inflammatory and analgesic properties, while stronger remedies such as turmeric, samambaia, milk thistle, or sarsaparilla address the underlying cause of the condition.

Diet's impact on skin health

A balanced diet is crucial to achieving beautiful, healthy, glowing skin, even though many of us are aware of how our food intake affects our waistlines.

Those who decide to alter their diet should be mindful of the potential effects on their skin, regardless of the reason for the change—weight loss or healthier eating choices.

The effects of specific meals on the skin:

Over time, consuming a diet high in processed foods, prepared meals, and refined carbs may lead to minor inflammation in the body and exacerbate skin conditions like acne.

Though most of us are aware of the damaging consequences of a poor diet on our skin, did you also know that food can help prevent the damaging effects of UV radiation from the sun on our skin?

Uv radiation exposure encourages the production of free radicals, which can harm the elastin and collagen that give our skin its structure and firmness. This can cause fine lines and wrinkles to become more noticeable over time!

How does this relate to your diet, then? Consuming foods high in antioxidants, such as vibrant fruits and vegetables, can help enhance the texture of the skin and prevent free radical damage.

Key food groups to be aware of which improve your skin – and which to avoid

Omega-3 fatty acids, which are known to improve skin health and reduce inflammation, are found in fish, making it a fantastic source of protein—essential for the formation of collagen and elastin, which keeps your skin supple.

Carotenoids, which are substances that are rich in color and give orange or red fruit and vegetables their color, can be turned into vitamin a, which is necessary for the regeneration of skin cells. They are also a fantastic source of vitamin C, which is necessary for the synthesis of collagen. Furthermore, because both carotenoids and vitamin C are antioxidants, they help fend against free radicals, which can harm our skin and prematurely age it.

Steer clear of processed carbohydrates and sugars, which include many breakfast cereals, candies, white bread, pastries, white rice, and sugary drinks. Replace these items with "good carbs" or meals high in antioxidants that prevent wrinkles, whole grains, and healthful veggies. Fruits also have a lower glycemic index. This will minimize the amount of carbohydrates in your diet overall.

It is imperative that your body gets adequate water when following a diet. It's critical to maintain hydration so that nutrients can get to the cells in your skin. Steer clear of sugar-filled beverages and sip on water or green tea instead, as these are excellent sources of antioxidants.

Your skin will reflect your dietary choices more strongly the healthier they are.

The resurgence of interest in herbal medicines offers a welcome alternative for individuals looking for a more natural approach to health and wellness in a world where modern medicine is taking over. Let's examine the importance of this manual and how it might enable people to care for their health naturally.

There are probably a lot of herbal goods on shelves when you walk into a health food store.

Herbs used medicinally are nothing new. They have actually been in use for millennia. They are now more commonly available to the general public, who may or may not be aware of their traditional applications.

Herbs are included in teas, meals, and cosmetics. Herbal skin treatments, sparkling herbal drinks, and herbal ghees are available.

They typically come in attractive packaging and are filled with alluring components like rhodiola rosea, lion's mane mushroom, and ashwagandha.

Do these herbal mixtures really have the therapeutic properties they promise? How can you choose which ones are best for you?

Mental health and stress relief

Everyone suffers stress, which is normal when they are faced with hazardous or dangerous situations. Your body reacts to stress by causing both physical and emotional side effects. Positive stress reactions can keep you motivated, aware of potential threats, and flexible in unfamiliar circumstances.

While stress by itself is not a disease, continuous exposure to it raises the possibility of developing mental health issues such as substance abuse issues, anxiety, depression, and psychosis.

Impact of stress on your mental health

The body can undergo minor to severe alterations as a result of stress. Cognitive, physical, emotional, or behavioral symptoms are all possible. Your body's autonomic nervous system takes over when you're under stress. The heart, stomach, and intestines are among the internal organs whose functions are governed by this system.

When you perceive danger, your muscles tense, your breathing and pulse rate quicken, your short-term memory sharpens, and your body gets ready for "fight or flight." stress levels and frequency can be beneficial or detrimental. When taken in moderation, it helps sharpen cognitive abilities and ease performance-related stress, such as that experienced during an exam. It can also help you become more adept in quick thinking, such as coming up with an instant solution to a problem.

Herbs for mood improvement and anxiety reduction

The effects of various plants on the body can vary.

For instance, ashwagandha has the ability to lower blood levels of the stress hormone cortisol. Anxiety can occur in people who are exposed to high levels of cortisol in the blood for an extended period of time.

Certain herbs can help promote relaxation by changing how the brain processes signals. For instance, valerian root extracts may modulate gamma-aminobutyric acid receptors in the brain, which may encourage relaxation and lessen sensations of anxiety. Thus, a lot of people say valerian root helps treat sleep disorders, including insomnia.

Ashwagandha

Ashwagandha, also known as withania somnifera, is a member of the "adaptogen" class of plants. Adaptogens have an impact on the hormones and systems that control an individual's stress reaction. The use of ashwagandha in traditional Indian medicine, or ayurvedic medicine, is rather old.

A modest 2019 study looked into ashwagandha's ability to reduce stress and anxiety. There were 58 individuals in the 8-week research who reported feeling stressed. One of three treatments—ashwagandha extract at doses of 250 mg or 600 mg per day or a placebo—was given to each participant at random.

Compared to the placebo group, the ashwagandha-taking individuals had lower cortisol levels. They had better-quality sleep as well.

Individuals who consumed 600 mg of ashwagandha reported a notable decrease in their stress levels. However, those who took the ashwagandha at a reduced dose did not report feeling less stressed.

Another modest 2019 trial gave 240 mg of ashwagandha or a placebo for 60 days to 60 individuals with mild anxiety. Certain anxiety scores were significantly reduced in those using the herb but not in others.

Chamomile

A flowering herb that resembles a daisy is chamomile. German and roman chamomile are the two varieties of chamomile that can be used medicinally.

The following are some ways that some people use chamomile to reduce stress and anxiety:

- Tea

- Extract

- Tablet

- Skin cream

The effectiveness and safety of chamomile as a long-term treatment for generalized anxiety disorder (gad) were examined in a small clinical experiment conducted in 2016.

For 12 weeks, 1,500 mg of chamomile was given to each of the 93 participants. After 26 weeks, some people kept taking chamomile, while others switched to a placebo. Researchers found that participants who switched to a placebo were not any less likely than those who stayed taking chamomile to experience a relapse of symptoms related to gad. When there was a relapse, the symptoms were not as bad.

Allergies to chamomile might happen to some people. Certain medications, such as the antirejection medication cyclosporine and the blood thinner warfarin, may interact with it.

It is crucial that anyone on medication consult their physician prior to ingesting chamomile drinks or supplements.

Valerian

Asia and Europe are the native habitats of the valerian plant, or valeriana officinalis. The root has been used for millennia to treat depression, anxiety, and sleep issues. The effects of valerian have only been the subject of a small number of excellent studies yet. According to the national center for complementary and integrative

health (NCCIH) trusted source, there is not enough data to say whether valerian can treat depression or anxiety.

According to studies, valerian is typically safe. The NCCIH does point out that there is no data about the safety or long-term usage of valerian in the following groups:

- Pregnant people

- Parents who are nursing

- Children under 3 years old

Lavender

A flowering plant in the mint family is lavender. People often use lavender to reduce anxiety and soothe tense muscles.

Lavender can be used as an essential oil or to prepare drinks.

Terpenes are substances found in lavender essential oil (LEO). Two of these terpenes, linalyl acetate and linalool, may have a relaxing impact on chemical receptors in the brain, according to a 2017 review article.

According to the review, LEO might be a useful short-term treatment for anxiety disorders. Studies on LEO's long-term consequences are, however, scarce.

Galphimia glauca

A species of plant native to Mexico is called galphimia glauca. People once used it as a sedative to lessen anxiety.

A 2018 review found encouraging evidence supporting g. Glauca as an anxiety therapy. Unfortunately, due to a shortage of plant material, medicinal companies have not fully utilized its potential.

Passionflower

There are about 550 species in the passiflora family of plants, including passionflowers. According to certain research, p. Incarnata, a specific species, may be useful in the treatment of anxiety, agitation, and restlessness.

P. Incarnata is available as a liquid tincture or as a tablet.

Kava kava

The shrub known as kava kava, or just kava, is indigenous to the pacific ocean's islands. Scientists refer to it as piper methysticum.

Kava might be useful in lowering tension and anxiety. Nonetheless, there have been documented instances of kava-containing products seriously harming the liver- trusted source. Before using kava, one should always speak with a doctor.

Stress management and relaxation practices

Particularly if you are ill, relaxation techniques can improve your quality of life and reduce the symptoms of stress. Learn how to relax on your own by doing some research.

One excellent method for managing stress is to practice relaxation techniques. Relaxation is more than just having a hobby or finding mental tranquility. It's a procedure that mitigates the negative impacts of stress on your body and mind. Finding ways to unwind can help you manage the stress of daily life. Additionally, these solutions can help with chronic stress or stress associated with other health issues, including pain and heart disease.

Relaxation techniques can help you, regardless of how well-managed your stress is currently. It's simple to pick up basic relaxation techniques. Relaxation methods are low-risk and frequently cost nothing. Additionally, they are portable.

Start by finding easy ways to unwind so that you may begin to reduce stress in your life and enhance your general health and well-being.

The relaxation methods listed below can assist you in inducing the relaxation response and lowering your stress levels.

1. **Pay attention to your breath**. You take long, slow, deep breaths in this easy-to- use, effective technique (also known as belly or abdominal breathing). You carefully detach your attention from distracting ideas and feelings as you breathe. People with eating problems can benefit most from breath concentration as it can help them focus on their body in a more positive way. Nonetheless, this method might not be suitable for people with medical conditions, including heart failure or respiratory disorders that make breathing difficult.

2. **Body scan.** This method combines progressive muscular relaxation with breath awareness. Deep breathing for a few minutes is followed by concentrating on one muscle group or area of the body at a time and mentally releasing any tension you may be experiencing physically. By doing a body scan, you can become more conscious of the mind-body link. This method might not work as well for you if you just underwent surgery that negatively impacts your body

image or if you have other issues related to your body image.

3. **Guided imagery.** Using this approach, you can help yourself relax and focus by visualizing relaxing pictures, places, or experiences. You can find recordings of peaceful scenes online and in free apps; just be sure to select images that are meaningful to you personally and that you find comforting. Although guided imagery can help you strengthen a positive self-image, it can be challenging for people who struggle to visualize things in their minds or who have intrusive ideas.

4. **Meditating with mindfulness.** In order to engage in this exercise, you need to choose a comfortable position, pay attention to your breathing, and keep your thoughts from wandering to the past or the future. In recent years, this type of meditation has grown in popularity. According to research, it might be beneficial for those who are depressed, anxious, or in pain.

5. **Tai chi, yoga, and qigong.** These three ancient disciplines consist of a series of postures or flowing movements combined with rhythmic breathing. These exercises' physical components provide a mental focus that can help you stop your mind from racing. They can also improve your balance and flexibility. However, these relaxing methods may be too difficult for you if you are not typically active, suffer from health issues, or have a severe or incapacitating disease. Consult your physician before beginning them.

BOOK 12:

Enhancing Immune Function

Enhancing immune function

Numerous goods and supplements make the promise to strengthen immunity. However, maintaining a strong immune system involves more than just ingesting a supplement containing a combination of vitamins and minerals in a tablet or powder form.

Your immune system functions within an extremely fine equilibrium. It must be intelligent and powerful enough to combat a wide range of ailments and infections without being overly powerful to the point of needless overreaction.

It is extremely precisely controlled to do this, responding to many inputs and internal body processes. Complex, as I mentioned.

However, there are things you can do to assist and ensure that your immune system has everything it needs to work at its best, whether it's fending off a cold, the flu, or covid-19, which don't entail consuming supplements.

These methods for developing and keeping a robust, healthy immune system are supported by science:

- Maintain a healthy diet
- Engage in regular exercise
- Hydrate, hydrate, hydrate
- Make sure you get enough rest
- Minimize stress

Boosting immunity with specific herbs and foods

The body's primary defense against infection, disease, and illness is the immune system. It is made up of an extensive network of cells, tissues, and organs that work together to coordinate the body's defenses against pathogens, viruses, and poisons that could endanger our health. The millions of protective white blood cells that scour the lymphatic and blood systems continuously alert for any suspicious signals of illness, are a key element of our immune system. Our immune system fights an illness once it is identified and retains the information for future use.

By giving the body the resources it needs to create a protective response and combat oxidative stress, such as antioxidants, phytonutrients, vitamins, minerals, and fiber, our diets can help strengthen our immune systems. The more variety, the better, so aim to incorporate a wide range of vibrant whole meals, fruits, and vegetables from the following list.

Blood oranges

Although other, more fashionable "superfoods" may garner more media attention than the humble orange, blood oranges are the true stars of the citrus family. With the same amount of vitamin C, they have five times the antioxidant activity of a typical orange. A daily glass of blood orange juice for seven days could help lower inflammation and increase blood antioxidant levels, according to research.

Greek yogurt

Probiotic-rich Greek yogurt has a higher protein content than conventional yogurt. According to a recent meta-analysis, individuals who consumed probiotic-rich foods on a daily basis were less likely to have a cold than those who did not.

Pomegranates

Polyphenols found in pomegranates can aid in treating and avoiding colds and coughs. Research has indicated that high concentrations of polyphenol antioxidants, such as those present in pomegranate juice, can shorten colds by up to 40%.

Brazil nuts

Selenium, a crucial mineral for preventing oxidative stress, is found in Brazil nuts. As selenium has also been demonstrated to aid in the body's defense against viral infections, consuming a few Brazil nuts daily as part of a meal or snack will help guarantee that the immune system has adequate selenium to remain robust.

Wild salmon

Zinc, which is abundant in wild salmon, has been shown to help lessen the symptoms of the common cold. It also contains many omega-3 fatty acids, which support improved immune cell function, viral infection prevention, and inflammation reduction.

Broccoli

According to research by the University of California, broccoli is a fantastic food to include in your diet if you want to avoid getting sick. It has been demonstrated that cruciferous vegetables, such as broccoli, can strengthen immunity due to a plant compound called sulforaphane, which activates antioxidant genes and enzymes in certain immune cells. By doing this, they lower the risk of disease by battling free radicals.

Green tea

For a good reason, green tea is often listed among the exceptionally healthy foods. Flavonoids are antioxidants with anti-inflammatory and immune-boosting qualities found in them. A study found that the antioxidant catechin, which is abundant in green tea, has strong antibacterial and antiviral properties and can eradicate the influenza virus and germs that cause colds.

Ginger

Ginger is considered one of the greatest foods for relieving a common cold. According to a review published in the International Journal of Preventative Medicine, ginger's strong anti-inflammatory qualities were a major factor in the root's ability to ward off the flu or cold.

Shallots

Shallots have up to six times the amount of polyphenols as certain regular onions. It all comes down to the amount of quercetin. Quercetin is a key component in the body's defense against disease-causing free radical damage.

Dark chocolate

Magnesium is a mineral found in dark chocolate that is essential for bolstering the immune system. Magnesium aids in the infections' attachment to lymphocytes, enabling the body to eliminate them. You receive the greatest benefits of magnesium and immune-boosting properties, so make sure you select very dark chocolate (80% cocoa or above).

Kiwi

One of the most nutrient-dense fruits in the world, kiwis have twice the vitamin C level of oranges and are packed with antioxidants like lutein and zeaxanthin! Numerous substances, such as fiber, vitamin C, carotenes, and polyphenols, have been demonstrated to support immune system performance; coincidentally, all of these are also present in kiwis.

Oregano

Numerous spices and herbs are well-known for their immune-stimulating and antibacterial qualities. One such herb that is worth using in your cuisine is oregano. It may be useful in treating bacterial infections because it contains essential oils, which are recognized for their antibacterial, antiviral, and antifungal qualities.

Sleep's role in immune health

The immune system is vitally supported by sleep. A well-balanced immune system with robust innate and adaptive immunity, an effective response to vaccinations, and less severe allergic reactions is made possible by getting enough hours of high-quality sleep.

On the other hand, severe sleep issues, such as sleep disorders like insomnia, sleep apnea, and disturbance of the circadian rhythm, can impair the immune system's ability to function normally.

Adaptive immunity, innate immunity, and sleep

Sleep is a vital time for our bodies to recover, and research suggests that it is essential for maintaining the strength of our immune systems. As a matter of fact, sleep supports both adaptive and innate immunity.

Researchers have discovered that specific immune system components become more active at night. For instance, cytokines linked to inflammation are produced at higher levels. Sleep and the body's internal 24-hour clock, known as circadian rhythm, appear to be the driving forces behind this activity.

This inflammatory response may aid in healing when someone is ill or injured, strengthening innate and adaptive immunity while the body heals wounds and fights off infections.

However, research has shown that this inflammation can happen even when a person is not physically ill or injured. Strengthening adaptive immunity is the function of this immunological activity that occurs at night, according to analysis of the cells and cytokines involved.

Research indicates that sleep enhances immunological memory, just as it can aid the brain in integrating learning and memory. Sleep enhances the immune system's memory of identifying and responding to harmful antigens through the interaction of immune system components.

Although the exact reason this process occurs while you sleep is unknown to experts, there are a few theories as to why it could be:

Breathing and muscular activity decrease while you sleep, which frees up energy for the immune system to carry out these vital functions.

The body has developed so that these processes occur during nightly sleep because the inflammation that occurs during sleep might impair mental and physical performance if it happens during waking hours.

The hormone melatonin, which is released during the night and promotes sleep, is effective in reducing the stress that can result from inflammation while you sleep.

Even while the immune system is working while you sleep, it's important to note that this process is self-regulating. The body's circadian clock reduces this inflammation when the sleep phase ends.

Thus, adequate, high-quality sleep contributes to the immune system's delicate balance, which is necessary for both innate immunity and adaptive immunity.

Vaccines and sleep

Research has unequivocally demonstrated the benefits of sleep for adaptive immunity, including how it enhances the effects of vaccinations.

Vaccines function by administering a deactivated or weakened antigen to the body, which sets up an immunological reaction. Immunizations successfully train the immune system to identify and combat that antigen in this way.

One major aspect that influences how effective immunizations are is sleep. Research on swine flu (h1n1) and hepatitis vaccines has shown that the body's immune response is weakened in individuals who don't sleep the night after getting vaccinated. This can sometimes reduce the vaccine's protection and potentially the need for a second dosage.

Although complete sleep deprivation was a part of those experiments, other research has indicated that persons who regularly miss at least seven hours of sleep have lower vaccine efficiency. Individuals who sleep poorly may not allow their body to form immune memory, which could prevent them from being immune even when they have received vaccinations.

Allergies and sleep

As the immune system overreacts to something that most individuals do not find harmful, allergies arise. There is mounting evidence that allergies and sleep are related.

According to recent studies, an individual's circadian rhythm has a role in controlling how their body reacts to allergens. The chance and intensity of allergic reactions may rise when the circadian cycle is disturbed.

Allergies have also been linked to sleep deprivation. According to one study, those who have peanut allergies are more likely to experience an allergy attack when they lack sleep, as it reduces the amount of peanut exposure needed to cause an allergy reaction by 45%.

BOOK 13:

Women's Health Essentials

Women's health: natural approaches

Adopting healthy behaviors is the greatest approach to fend off illness, extend your life, and lead a happier existence. Nonetheless, a woman's hectic daily schedule, job, errands, and other commitments may take precedence over leading a healthy lifestyle.

Women have particular challenges when it comes to healthcare.

Naturopathic remedies can help with anything from painful periods to menopause, frequent yeast infections, to problems with fertility.

Natural management of menstrual and menopausal symptoms

The symptoms of menopause may persist for several months or even years. Women may experience distinct symptoms, such as:

- Irregular periods

- Vasomotor symptoms (VMS) - night sweats and hot flashes

- Vaginal dryness

- Chills

- Problems sleeping

- Mood problems

- Weight gain

- Hair or skin changes

- Loss of breast fullness

As an alternative to hormone replacement treatment, some women choose to treat their VMS using nutritional supplements and herbs. Menopausal symptoms can be treated naturally in a variety of ways.

Herbs for menopause symptom management

Although numerous herbs are well-liked, these are the most often utilized ones for menopause:

Black cohosh.

One of the most well-known herbs for treating menopause symptoms is black cohosh. Studies indicate that the active ingredients, triterpenoid isolates, and n- methylserotonin, may function as partial agonists of gaba and serotonin receptors. The advantages of mood and hot flashes may be explained by this interaction. Standard dosages (20–40 mg) have also been associated with a decrease in anxiety and depression in women going through menopause and perimenopause.

Red clover

Because of its isoflavone concentration, red clover is another herb that is frequently used to treat menopause-related symptoms. Plant substances called isoflavones replicate the physiological effects of estrogen. Red clover may help menopausal women feel better overall and experience fewer, milder hot flashes. This has been reported by a number of research.

Dong Quai

In traditional Chinese medicine, dong quai has been used extensively to treat menopause symptoms and balance hormones. However, there is scant and conflicting scientific data to support its efficacy. When combined with other herbs, dong quai has been shown in certain trials to help reduce menopause symptoms; however, further research is required to validate its safety and benefits.

Sage

Sage is thought to lessen a few menopause-related symptoms, like night sweats. Sage is thought to help control body temperature and lessen excessive perspiration. Additionally, sage contains antioxidants that may help guard against excessive inflammation and oxidative stress.

John's wort

Menopausal depression and mood swings are frequently treated with St. John's wort. St. John's wort is thought to help elevate serotonin and other neurotransmitter levels, which can alleviate depression. However, it is important to speak with a healthcare professional before using St. John's wort as it may interact with some drugs, such as blood thinners, birth control pills, and antidepressants.

Herbs that can be used to support fertility

Ashwagandha

In Ayurveda, ashwagandha (withania somnifera) is traditionally used to treat infertility and male sexual dysfunction. Since it is a calming adaptogen, people with nervous weariness, tension, and anxiety can benefit most from it. It is regarded as a revitalizing tonic for the neurological and reproductive systems. It's a nutritious herb that boosts sexual desire.

Damian

Damiana, or turnera diffusa, has long been used as a tonic for depression and nervous weariness, as well as a treatment for sexual dysfunction. It can assist in addressing low estrogen levels in women as well as help males manage their testosterone levels.

Lady's mantle

Ladies' mantle (alchemilla vulgaris) is frequently used to treat a variety of menstruation issues. It softly fortifies the uterine tissues and aids in the reduction of heavy monthly bleeding. It can aid in the promotion of conception and may enhance progesterone activity.

Shatavari

In ancient Ayurvedic medicine, shatavari (asparagus racemosus) is widely valued as a great reproductive tonic that supports healthy fertility. It can be used to treat any menstrual issues, prevent early miscarriage, increase sperm production in men, and lessen uterine contractions in women. It's a fantastic aphrodisiac as well!

Maca

The Andes mountain herb maca, also known as maca root, is a superfood and adaptogenic herb that is free of caffeine. Many people still use it now, having historically eaten it as a healthful food among the local people of the high-altitude Andes regions.

Apart from promoting mood, vitality, and a balanced stress reaction, maca is regarded as an aphrodisiac, which implies that it enhances the desire for sex. That's not all, though. The potential effect of maca on sperm is another potential reproductive advantage.

Maca was reported to boost sperm count and motility in a small trial involving nine healthy men.

Although further investigation and clinical trials are necessary to establish firm conclusions regarding the impact of this herb on enhanced sperm function, these encouraging preliminary findings excite us. Please be aware that the results of this study might not apply to your particular circumstance;

therefore, you should always see your doctor before beginning any new treatment.

BOOK 14:

Chronic Inflammation and

Cancer Prevention

Combating chronic inflammation

Though it's invisible to the naked eye, inflammation may be gradually harming your health.

As part of the body's natural healing process, inflammation (swelling) aids in the body's defense against injury and infection. However, it doesn't only occur in reaction to disease and trauma. When the immune system activates in the absence of damage or illness to combat, an inflammatory response may also result. The immune system cells that typically defend us start to kill good arteries, organs, and joints because there is nothing to mend.

Varinthrej Pitis, MD, an internal medicine specialist at Scripps Clinic Carmel Valley, states that the body reacts by producing inflammation when you don't eat healthily, don't exercise enough, or experience too much stress. "Over time, chronic inflammation might have detrimental effects. Therefore, when it comes to lowering inflammation, what you eat, how well you sleep, and how much you exercise are all actually important.

What does chronic inflammation do to the body?

Chronic inflammation might have hazy early symptoms, with mild indications and symptoms that could go unnoticed for a very long time. It could be that you're just a little tired, or that's normal. However, as inflammation worsens, it starts to harm your joints, organs, and arteries. If neglected, it can exacerbate long-term health issues like diabetes, obesity, cancer, heart disease, blood vessel disease, alzheimer's disease, and other ailments.

Fatty deposits in the artery lining of the heart are a result of immune system cells that inflame the tissue. These plaques have the potential to burst at some point, forming a clot that may obstruct an artery. Heart attacks are the outcome of obstruction.

The most popular method of measuring inflammation is to perform a blood test for the inflammatory marker hs-crp, or c-reactive protein. Homocysteine levels are another indicator used by doctors to assess chronic inflammation. Lastly, to evaluate damage to red blood cells, doctors check for blood sugar levels using the hba1c test.

Anti-inflammatory diet and lifestyle adjustments

Anti-inflammatory diets are usually eating habits rather than regimens. Two anti- inflammatory diets are the dash diet and the Mediterranean diet.

In many circumstances, dietary modifications can help manage inflammation—both short- and long-term—although their effectiveness as a management strategy will rely on the individual's general health and the underlying causes of the inflammation. For instance, psoriasis, rheumatoid arthritis, and asthma can all result in persistent inflammation. While altering one's diet may help control some symptoms, it may not be helpful in more severe situations.

Certain foods have components that can either cause or exacerbate inflammation. Conversely, certain foods have ingredients like antioxidants that may actually lessen it.

Antioxidants' function

The mainstay of an anti-inflammatory diet is fresh produce, which is rich in antioxidants.

Foods contain compounds known as dietary antioxidants that aid in the body's elimination of free radicals.

Naturally occurring byproducts of several body functions, such as metabolism, are free radicals. Cell damage may result from free radicals. This damage can lead to a number of disorders and raises the risk of inflammation.

Antioxidant-rich meals are preferred over foods that boost the formation of free radicals in an anti-inflammatory diet.

Oily fish, which is high in omega-3 fatty acids, may help lower the body's levels of inflammatory proteins. Fiber may also provide this outcome.

Types of anti-inflammatory diet

Anti-inflammatory concepts are already included in several well-known diets. For example, fresh fruits and vegetables, seafood, whole grains, and heart-healthy fats are all part of the Mediterranean diet and the dietary approaches to stop hypertension (dash) diet.

For instance, studies indicate that the Mediterranean diet, which emphasizes plant- based foods and healthy fats, may help lessen the negative effects of inflammation on the heart.

Additionally, compared to conventional diets, studies indicate that the dash diet may be beneficial in lowering markers of inflammation. In inflammatory arthritis disorders, the dash diet may also have other advantages, such as reducing uric acid levels, which are a risk factor for gout.

Foods to eat

A varied diet high in nutrients should be a part of any anti-inflammatory plan.

- Provides a range of antioxidants.

- Contains healthful fats.

Some foods that could assist in reducing inflammation are:

- Oily fish, such as tuna and salmon

- Fruits, such as blueberries, blackberries, strawberries, and cherries

- Vegetables, including kale, spinach, and broccoli

- Beans

- Nuts and seeds

- Olives and olive oil

- Fiber

- Raw or moderately cooked vegetables

- Legumes, such as lentils

- Spices such as ginger and turmeric

- Probiotics and prebiotics

- Tea

- Some herbs

It's important to keep in mind that no single food can improve one's health. It is crucial to incorporate a range of nutritious foods into the diet.

Foods to limit

Processed foods are something that people on an anti-inflammatory diet should stay away from or consume in moderation.

- Foods that have salt or sugar added.

- Unhealthy oils.

- Processed carbohydrates found in many baked items, white bread, and white pasta.

- Processed foods for snacks, including crackers and chips.

- Prepared sweets, including ice cream, candies, and cookies.

- Overindulgence in alcohol.

Additionally, some people may be intolerant to particular foods, which means that consuming them can have negative effects like inflammation. Typical intolerances consist of:

- Gluten

- Dairy

- Nightshade vegetables

- Cruciferous vegetables

Steps to an anti-inflammatory lifestyle

You'll be relieved to hear that adopting an anti-inflammatory lifestyle is simpler than you might think if you believe you are susceptible to chronic inflammation and all of its terrible effects. You can lessen your inflammation and keep it from worsening by following these easy tips.

Fight inflammation with genuine food: many delectable options on the menu are available to help reduce inflammation. By removing harmful byproducts or preventing specific phases of the inflammatory cascade, eating the correct nutrients can support your body.

Antioxidants are abundant in the finest meals that reduce inflammation. Antioxidants have a powerful anti-inflammatory effect because they bind to and neutralize dangerous "oxygen free radicals," which are byproducts of inflammation. This effectively halts oxidative damage.

Try the anti-inflammatory spice, turmeric. Recently, certain specific substances have gained attention as powerful anti-inflammatory agents. Turmeric, for instance, has established a strong reputation for lowering inflammation linked to cancer, arthritis, and alzheimer's disease.

Curcumin in turmeric suppresses inflammation by lowering free radical levels and inhibiting pro-inflammatory indicators. You can ingest turmeric in food, as a tea, in capsule form, or as a solution.

Eliminate the chemicals: pesticides and preservatives promote inflammation by infiltrating cells and damaging tissue. These substances also significantly impact our gut flora, which functions as an additional immune system. This vital layer of defense is destroyed by repeated exposure, which results in more tissue loss and inflammation.

Take extra care when using cleaning supplies. Many natural alternatives work well and are far less harmful to you and your family. When it comes to toothpaste, shampoo, cosmetics, and other personal hygiene items, carefully read the labels. Steer clear of parabens and phthalates at all costs.

Making healthier dietary choices can also help you limit your exposure to chemicals. Try to consume seasonal, local, and ideally organic food when possible. If this isn't possible, make sure to thoroughly wash your veggies. Choose home-cooked meals over highly processed ones that are packaged in plastic.

Take pleasure in exercising: frequent exercise successfully lowers inflammation by enhancing lymphatic and circulatory flow, decreasing body fat, and increasing circulation. Any kind of exercise will do as long as it raises your heart rate. Make it a goal to work out five days a week for at least thirty minutes, and gradually increase your time.

It is crucial to maintain a healthy weight in order to counteract inflammation. Obesity puts the body under metabolic stress, which can cause fat cells to contribute to the initiation of an inflammatory response. This occurs because fat cells have the ability to release cytokines, which stimulate immune cells to start an inflammatory response, making them behave like immune cells.

Make getting enough sleep a genuine priority. If I could recommend one healthy habit for my patients to adopt on their own, it would be to make creating a sleep routine a top priority and stick to it religiously. Your body may heal from the mental and physical stresses of the day while you sleep. That recovery period is severely shortened by interrupted, poor-quality sleep.

It's alluring to stay up late working or scrolling through social media. Treat yourself well, retire to bed at a respectable hour, and maintain a cool, cozy, and dark environment in your room. Take the phone and tv out of the bedroom and give yourself some time to relax and be still. Melatonin is a natural sleep hormone that supports a healthy circadian rhythm. If you have difficulties falling asleep, you might want to think about taking a supplement.

Modify how you react to stress: anxiety and stress can also cause inflammation. Regardless of the source, the body perceives these feelings as internal intruders and generates inflammatory signals all over the body to stave against oncoming harm.

The likelihood that you may experience inflammation increases with the amount of stress in your life. Both journaling and beginning a meditation program are great ways to relieve tension every night. There are countless ways to reduce stress, so try a few different approaches until you find the one that works for you if the first one doesn't seem like it will work for you.

Recall that you don't need to implement each of these adjustments right now. Choose one to begin with, and then add another once it becomes a habit.

Herbal anti-inflammatories and their usage.

Certain herbal medicines contain natural chemicals that may also have anti- inflammatory properties. Still, very little research has been done in this field.

- Turmeric

- Ginger

- Green tea

Anti-inflammatory qualities may also be present in many other herbal medicines. For example, consider:

- Thyme

- White willow bark

- Frankincense

- Resveratrol

Cancer prevention and support

How may one reduce their risk of developing cancer? There's no shortage of counsel. However, recommendations from different studies can conflict with one another. Information on cancer prevention is still being developed. It is widely acknowledged, nevertheless, that lifestyle decisions have an impact on cancer risk.

As part of breast cancer awareness month, an annual effort aimed at raising awareness and money, people worldwide wear pink attire in October. These initiatives help fund research that could save lives and offer individuals impacted life- altering assistance. Powerful tales of resiliency abound during this season, reminding us of the struggles many people endure in the face of this difficult illness.

However, the topic of discussion goes beyond breast cancer. It's important to keep in mind that cancer takes many different forms and affects many people and their families in ways that go beyond just one month and one type of disease. There's a larger conversation about cancer awareness and prevention than just the October stories and symbols. As we examine this crucial subject, it becomes evident that the greatest ways for us to stop this illness are through education and teamwork.

Each component of our complex systems depends on and links to the others. When we mention cancer, we're talking about a disruption in this system that's frequently brought on by lifestyle choices, the environment, and genetics. Every decision we make, from what we eat to how frequently we exercise, has the power to strengthen or weaken our defenses.

Our daily choices, which we frequently make without giving them much attention, have a significant impact on both our risk of cancer and our general health. For example, the foods we choose to eat can have a significant role in preventing cancer. Consuming a diet high in fruits, vegetables, and whole grains gives you vital nutrients and antioxidants that fight the chemicals that cause cancer. Conversely, consuming red meats, processed foods, and foods heavy in sugar and bad fats on a regular basis can increase our risk.

Likewise, maintaining our physical fitness and controlling our weight are not the only goals of our exercise levels. Frequent exercise guarantees effective blood circulation bolsters the immune system and supports gut health—all of which are critical in preventing cancer. On the other hand, a sedentary lifestyle—one that involves extended periods of inactivity—can increase our susceptibility to many cancers.

Every decision we make about our diet, exercise routine, or even stress management builds upon the other, either fortifying or, regrettably, weakening our body's defenses against cancer. Being aware of these variables and their effects is essential to taking a proactive stance in cancer prevention. Let's investigate these elements more thoroughly and find practical solutions to strengthen our resistance against cancer.

Foods that prevent cancer

Mushrooms and immune-boosting foods.

For a long time, people have valued mushrooms for their therapeutic qualities in addition to their culinary appeal. Some types are particularly notable for having potential anti-cancer properties; experts such as Dr. Andrew Weil has frequently emphasized these. For example, lentinan, a substance found in shiitake mushrooms, has been demonstrated to boost immunity and inhibit the growth of cancer cells. Further research has been done on the immune-stimulating and anti-cancer effects of maitake, reishi, and lion's mane mushrooms. Including these mushrooms in our diet can be a tasty and advantageous approach to take advantage of their health- enhancing properties.

Other foods besides mushrooms have also shown promise in bolstering the body's anti-cancer defenses. Numerous studies have connected green tea, which is high in the antioxidants called catechins, to a lower risk of cancer. Frequent consumption of it can aid the body's defense against dangerous free radicals. Strawberries, raspberries, and blueberries are just a few of the berries that are rich in antioxidants, fiber, and vitamins. These little fruits have a big potential to stop cell damage that could cause cancer. We're strengthening our body's natural defenses and satisfying our taste buds at the same time when we include these foods in our regular meals.

Nutrient-rich foods.

The Mediterranean diet, widely regarded as one of the world's healthiest eating plans, is a well-balanced combination of flavor and health advantages. This diet, which has its roots in the customs of Mediterranean-coastal nations, places a strong emphasis on whole grains, fresh produce, lean meats like shellfish and fish, and heart-healthy fats like olive oil. A mainstay of this diet is seafood, especially fatty fish like sardines, mackerel, and salmon. These fish are high in omega-3 fatty acids, which have been connected to a lower risk of developing a number of cancers. Later on, more on this. Complete grains, like quinoa, offer vital fiber that promotes healthy digestion and lowers the risk of colorectal cancer. Legumes, such as chickpeas and lentils, are high in protein and also contain a lot of antioxidants and phytochemicals that can slow the formation of cancer. Then there are the unsung heroes of the food world, like Brazil nuts, which are rich in selenium, a potent antioxidant that may lower the chance of developing several types of cancer. Adopting a Mediterranean diet not only provides us with a delicious meal, but it also gives our bodies the nourishment they require to fight cancer.

The power of vegetables.

Vegetables are nature's method of providing us with a protective barrier for our health, with their vivid colors and varied textures. However, their advantages go beyond simply making our meals seem pretty. Every shade and variation have their own special combination of nutrients and chemicals that help prevent cancer. Brussels sprouts, kale, broccoli, and cauliflower are among the superfoods known as cruciferous vegetables. They contain a lot of glucosinolates, which have been demonstrated to inhibit the growth of tumors and lower the chance of developing some types of cancer.

Allicin, a substance with possible anti-cancer effects, is found in garlic and is a staple in many cuisines. Frequent garlic consumption has been associated with a lower risk of cancer, particularly stomach and colon cancers. On the other hand, lycopene, an antioxidant with potential protection against prostate cancer, is abundant in tomatoes.

We are improving more than just the taste and appearance of our meals when we make sure that our vegetable consumption is varied and vibrant. By actively utilizing these veggies' anti-cancer properties, we're equipping our bodies with the strongest natural defenses against cancer.

Seeds with omega-3 fatty acids.

Due to their well-known ability to reduce inflammation, omega-3 fatty acids are essential in the battle against cancer. These necessary fats have been connected to a lower incidence of prostate, colon, and breast cancers, among other cancers. These healthy fats are mostly found in the Mediterranean diet, but supplements are another good source for people who may not eat fish frequently.

The advantages of omega-3s are enhanced by seeds, especially flaxseeds. These little powerhouses of nourishment are loaded with lignans, fiber, and a healthy serving of omega-3 fatty acids. The combination of these minerals found in flaxseeds has been linked to a lower risk of cancer, particularly colon and breast cancer. One simple way to add ground flaxseeds' health benefits to our diet is to consume them in smoothies, oatmeal, or baked goods.

We are proactively strengthening our body's defenses against potential cancer risks by emphasizing our intake of omega-3 fatty acids and including seeds like flaxseeds in our meals.

Nature's pharmacists

Spices have been valued for their therapeutic qualities as well as for culinary contributions throughout history. Turmeric is a standout in this category because of its vivid golden color. It's a powerful ally for health and a common ingredient in many recipes. Curcumin, the main ingredient in turmeric, has been the subject of much research due to its potential anti-inflammatory and antioxidant effects. According to research, curcumin may even be able to stop cancer cells from ever starting in the first place.

No other spices have the same powerful health effects as turmeric. Grapes are more than simply a delicious snack; they're also a popular ingredient in wines. They are particularly high in the potent antioxidant resveratrol, especially the red and purple types. Numerous anti-cancer effects of resveratrol have been demonstrated, ranging from preventing cancer cells from proliferating to actually killing them.

We're doing more than just enhancing the taste and texture of our meals when we include these "natural pharmacists" in our regular diet. We are drawing on age-old wisdom by utilizing the therapeutic and preventive qualities of these spices and adding an additional layer of defense to our bodies against cancer.

Exercise for cancer prevention

Exercise frequently conjures images of lean muscles, heightened endurance, or even weight loss. However, the advantages of consistent exercise go far beyond the scale and the mirror. All forms of movement are powerful tools in our fight against cancer. Whether it's a vigorous workout, a yoga class, or a brisk walk, you're accomplishing more than just burning calories and developing strength when you move your body. By doing this, you are actively strengthening your body's defenses against possible health hazards.

Our immune systems can be revitalized by exercise, which is one of its amazing advantages. Our first line of defense is a strong immune system that is constantly scanning the body for rogue cells that may develop into cancer. We guarantee the continued vigilance and sharpness of this protection mechanism by staying engaged. Exercise is also essential for the control of hormones. Hormonal abnormalities have been connected to a number of diseases, including prostate and breast cancer. Frequent exercise lowers the risk of cancer by maintaining a healthy balance of these hormones. Additionally, exercise indirectly reduces the incidence of malignancies connected to obesity by helping with weight management. Not to be overlooked is the part exercise plays in detoxifying. By helping our bodies get rid of pollutants, sweating it out can help lower the risk of cancer.

Thus, keep in mind the significant benefits of movement for your health the next time you're debating missing that workout or choosing the elevator over the stairs. Every move made and every rep finished counts as a step toward a future free from cancer.

Easing migraines and headaches

If you have migraines or headaches frequently, you might be wondering if there's a method to avoid them or what will help ease your pain and other symptoms when you do. Are there any steps you may take on your own, even if your doctor has prescribed medicine or other treatments?

Yes, is the response. When used in conjunction with doctor-prescribed therapy, home remedies, and lifestyle modifications can have an additive effect, even if they may not be able to prevent or relieve all headaches or migraine attacks.

It may be easier to determine what kinds of natural and home treatments could prevent headaches and migraine attacks if you know what causes or triggers them. According to Medlineplus, tension headaches are produced by tense muscles in the shoulders, neck, scalp, and jaw, which can be brought on by stress, depression, anxiety, and exhaustion. According to the World Health Organization, tension headaches impact over half of women and over a third of men in industrialized nations, and they are also becoming more common in developing nations (who).

According to the National Headache Foundation, 13 percent of Americans experience migraine attacks, which are more than twice as common in women as in males. The American Migraine Foundation states that weather variations, exhaustion, stress, worry, lack of sleep, dehydration, and hormonal fluctuations (in women) can all cause migraines. Other triggers for an attack include fasting, traveling to a higher altitude, traveling without eating, and, for certain people, consuming alcohol or the dietary ingredient monosodium glutamate (MSG).

According to Jennifer Kriegler, MD, a neurologist and former chairman of the Cleveland Clinic's

Headache Medicine Fellowship in Ohio, you should always see your doctor before attempting any complementary therapies or supplements to treat migraine episodes or headaches.

According to Dr. Kriegler, "Even natural substances have side effects." In addition, "What you believe you're buying isn't always what you get" is a problem with dietary and herbal supplements since they aren't subject to FDA regulation in the United States.

Natural preventative measures for migraines and headaches

The same lifestyle decisions supporting general health can also help you have fewer migraines and less pain.

The most successful strategy to manage migraines is frequently to combine medication with lifestyle changes and behavioral therapies.

Find a peaceful setting

If you can, stop what you're doing and take a break as soon as you feel the beginnings of a migraine. Switch off the lights. Migraine discomfort may worsen in response to light and music. Unwind in a peaceful, dark room. If you can, go to sleep.

Sleep well

Migraines may hinder your ability to fall asleep or stay asleep at night. Similarly, inadequate sleep is often the cause of migraines.

Eat wisely

Your migraines may be influenced by the food you eat. Think about the fundamentals: Maintain consistency. Every day, eat at roughly the same hour. Never miss a meal. Migraine risk rises with fasting.

Maintain a food diary. It can be helpful to identify possible dietary triggers by keeping a journal of the things you eat and the times you get migraines.

Engage in regular exercise

Your body releases particular chemicals when you exercise, which prevent your brain from receiving pain signals. These substances also aid in the reduction of depression and anxiety, two states that can exacerbate migraines.

Manage stress

Migraines and stress frequently coexist. Although daily stress is unavoidable, it can be managed to help with migraine management:

BOOK 15:

Treatments for Cold, Allergy,

and Men's Health

Natural remedies for the common cold and flu

Fever, fatigue, and chills are some of the symptoms that may accompany a flu infection. There is no known cure for the flu, although some of its symptoms may be eased with natural and household remedies.

A virus causes influenza, sometimes known as the flu. The flu can be caused by a variety of viruses. Although there isn't a cure for the flu, there are several natural treatments that could lessen its effects. They might also aid in reducing the duration of your flu.

Consume liquids, especially water

It is even more crucial to stay hydrated when suffering from the illness. This is true whether you get the stomach flu or the respiratory flu.

Drinking water keeps your throat, mouth, and nose wet. This aids in the body's removal of mucus and phlegm accumulation.

Dehydration can also occur if you aren't eating or drinking regularly. Water loss is also a common side effect of fever and diarrhea, two common flu symptoms.

To stay hydrated, be sure to eat lots of:

- Water

- Coconut water

- Sports drinks

- Herbal tea

- Fresh juice

- Soup

- Broth

- Raw fruits and vegetables

If you routinely need to urinate, then you're probably getting enough water and other liquids in your diet.

Your pee has a light yellow or nearly clear color.

You can be dehydrated if the color of your urine is dark yellow to amber.

Smoking should also be avoided as much as possible as it might aggravate your throat, lungs, and nose.

Get enough sleep

When you have the flu, it's crucial to rest and sleep more. Resting can strengthen your defenses against illness. This aids in the body's defense against the flu virus. To help you get back on your feet, stop your regular schedule and prioritize getting enough sleep.

Sip on some heated broth

You can stay hydrated by consuming warm bone broth, such as that made from chicken or cattle. It aids in clearing out sinus and nasal congestion.

Additionally, bone broth is naturally high in protein and minerals like potassium and salt. While you're sick with the flu, drinking broth is a smart way to replace these minerals. Moreover, protein is necessary for the regeneration of immunological cells. You can purchase premade versions, but make sure to choose ones with less sodium (salt). Boiling chicken or cow bones will yield a homemade broth. Broth can be frozen in parts for later use.

Sip on some herbal tea

Numerous herbs possess inherent antiviral and antibacterial qualities. Oseltamivir was historically derived from star anise, a spice shaped like a star.

Prescription medication oseltamivir phosphate, popularly known as tamiflu, is used to either prevent or treat influenza. Certain types of flu viruses can be effectively combatted by their antiviral characteristics. Antioxidant and antibacterial properties are also found in other herbs and green leafy teas.

Having a herbal tea could aid your body in warding off the flu. Your sinuses and throat will also feel better after drinking a hot herbal tea.

Star anise can be combined with other herbs to form a herbal drink that fights the flu.

- Green or black tea

- Turmeric

- Fresh or dried ginger or ginger paste

- Fresh garlic

- Cloves

Use pure honey to sweeten herbal teas. Natural antiviral and antibacterial qualities have been discovered in honey, royal jelly, and other bee products.

You can find these as dried components blended in a lot of bagged teas.

Men's health: prostate support and vitality

In the fast-paced metropolis of New York, where time seems to stand still, it is crucial to take responsibility for our well-being. Men's health sometimes goes unnoticed, yet the prostate is a little gland that plays a big part in general wellbeing. It can be difficult to maintain a healthy prostate as we age, but with the correct techniques, we can guarantee that this important organ continues to perform at its best.

Recognizing the prostate and its difficulties

The prostate, a walnut-sized gland beneath the bladder, is essential to the health of male reproduction. Men are more likely to develop prostate problems as they age, including benign prostatic hyperplasia (BPH) and prostate cancer. If left untreated, symptoms can include poor urine flow and frequent urination, as well as more catastrophic consequences. The good news is that you can successfully and naturally promote the health of your prostate by taking a proactive approach.

Natural ingredients for prostate health

In order to promote the health of their prostate, many men have resorted to natural components. They have discovered that these cures operate in perfect harmony to preserve and enhance their well-being. Let's investigate a few of these natural treasures and hear from people who have profited from using them.

Saw palmetto

Saw palmetto has long been used to promote prostate health; it is derived from the berries of the serenoa repens plant. Because of its capacity to lessen BPH symptoms, it is widely used in natural health circles.

Shilajit

Shilajit is a naturally occurring substance that is abundant in fulvic acid and minerals and is mostly found in the rocks of the Himalayas. Ayurvedic medicine has long been used to maintain general health, particularly prostate function, and increase energy.

Pomegranate extract

Pomegranate extract has anti-inflammatory and antioxidant qualities. It is made from the nutrient-rich seeds of the pomegranate fruit. According to studies, it can help lower PSA (prostate-specific antigen) levels and delay the onset of prostate problems.

Iodine

In addition to being vital for thyroid function, iodine is also important for prostate health. By promoting hormonal balance, adequate iodine levels can help lower the likelihood of prostate issues.

Lifestyle changes for prostate health

A healthy prostate requires not just these natural nutrients but also a lifestyle change. Prostate health can be enhanced by regular exercise, a balanced diet rich in fruits and vegetables, drinking enough water, and limiting alcohol and caffeine.

Frequent checks: the secret to preventive health

It's critical to combine routine medical checkups with lifestyle modifications and natural therapies.

Potential problems can be identified early on with screenings like PSA testing, preventing them from getting worse. Speaking with a healthcare professional guarantees that you are headed in the correct direction and enables you to receive individualized guidance based on your unique requirements.

Exercise and stress reduction for overall vitality

Engaging in physical activity not only extends your life but also improves it. It can prevent a variety of ailments, strengthen your heart and muscles, enhance your mental and emotional well-being, increase productivity, and strengthen your bonds with others. Continue reading to learn five ways that exercise can raise your standard of living.

1. **Prevents depression:** although a few laps around the block won't address major emotional problems, regular exercise has been shown to be strongly associated with happier moods, according to a study. Stress-relieving and wellbeing-enhancing hormones are released when aerobic exercise is performed. Furthermore, practically all forms of exercise involve rhythmic muscular contractions that raise serotonin levels in the brain, a neurotransmitter that helps fight off depressive symptoms.

2. **Improves sex life:** moderate to intense aerobic exercise increases libido and performance. According to the Harvard Health Professionals follow-up study, men who worked out for thirty minutes a day had a 41% lower risk of erectile dysfunction than men who did not exercise. Women also benefit from exercise: a research found that 20 minutes of cycling increased women's sexual arousal by 169%.

3. **Sharpens wits:** exercise increases cerebral blood flow, which may support cognitive health. Additionally, it supports healthy lung function, which is a quality shared by those whose mental clarity and memory hold up well into old age. While physical activity of any kind

keeps the mind active, numerous studies have demonstrated that aerobic exercise specifically enhances cognitive function.

4. **Enhances sleep:** engaging in regular aerobic exercise helps you sleep better by promoting quicker sleep, longer deep sleep, and fewer nighttime awakenings. The only known method for healthy adults to increase their deep sleep is through exercise, and deep sleep is necessary for your body to mend and rejuvenate itself.

5. **Preserves vigor and mobility:** frequent exercise helps mitigate the aging-related natural loss in physical performance. In fact, older folks can maintain muscular function, metabolism, and cardiovascular fitness levels comparable to those of far younger people by maintaining an active lifestyle. More research has also revealed that those who maintained greater levels of activity throughout their middle years were able to maintain their mobility and, consequently, their independence as they became older.

Allergy relief and management

Your body reacts to foreign proteins with allergies. These proteins, or allergens, are usually safe. On the other hand, your body's immune system overreacts to the presence of a protein if you have an allergy to it.

What is an allergic reaction?

Your body's reaction to an allergen is called an allergic reaction.

When an allergy sufferer comes into contact with a particular allergen for the first time, their body produces immunoglobulin E (IGE). To create IGE, your immune system produces antibodies.

The mast cells (allergy cells) in your skin, respiratory tract (airways), and mucous membrane in the hollow organs from your mouth to your anus (gastrointestinal or gi tract) are all bound by IGE antibodies.

By carrying the allergens to the mast cell, also known as the allergy cell, where they bind to a specific receptor, the antibodies locate the allergens in your body and aid in their elimination. The allergy cell releases histamine as a result of this. The culprit behind your allergy symptoms is histamine.

How common are allergies?

Allergies occur frequently.

Every year in the us, allergic reactions affect over 50 million people. In the us, they rank as the sixth most common cause of chronic illness.

Who is affected by allergies?

Anybody can be impacted by allergies.

If either of your biological parents has allergies, you have a higher chance of developing allergies as well.

Foods that may help curb your allergies

Do you find seasonal sneezes, itches, and sniffles bothersome? You can eat some foods that can help reduce the symptoms of your allergies.

There is no known nutritional remedy. However, fruits and vegetables are beneficial to your entire body. They are nutrient-rich and can help you stay well. Additionally, they might shield you from seasonal allergies.

Try these things:

Quercetin is found in berries, parsley, onions, and peppers. Quercetin is a naturally occurring plant compound, according to integrative medicine specialist Elson Haas, MD. Haas claims that this substance might lessen "histamine responses." One component of the allergic reaction is histamine.

Kiwi is a fuzzy, vitamin C-rich fruit. Histamine levels can also be reduced by it. Numerous foods, particularly oranges and other citrus fruits, are good sources of vitamin C.

Bromelain is an enzyme found in pineapples. Bromelain helps lessen irritation in allergic illnesses like asthma, claims Lawrence Rosen, MD.

Omega-3 fatty acids are found in mackerel, salmon, and tuna. Omega-3 has anti-inflammatory properties. Aim for two servings each week of fish. According to a Japanese study, women with higher fish intakes experienced less hay fever or allergic rhinitis.

Kefir is a probiotic-rich yogurt beverage. These are beneficial bacteria that reside in your digestive system. Rosen claims that they might even be able to treat and prevent seasonal allergies. Probiotics are present in fermented foods. On the label, look for yogurts that state "live active cultures." kimchi and sauerkraut are other excellent sources.

Local honey. The study is conflicting regarding whether using local honey prevents allergies. Rosen warns that if you consume small amounts of honey early in the season, you can become tolerant to the pollen in your area. According to one study, those who consumed birch pollen honey experienced fewer birch pollen allergy symptoms than those who consumed normal honey. While it's not guaranteed, give it a try.

Diet changes to reduce seasonal allergies

For those who suffer from allergies, a shift in the weather might result in a major adjustment to their way of life, such as experimenting with at-home treatments or over-the-counter medications and completely avoiding some environments. Thankfully, you won't have to go through allergy season irritations this year. This season, get ahead of your allergies by paying attention to these everyday health dietary recommendations.

Take a cup of green tea every morning

It has been demonstrated that the beverage's natural antihistamines lessen allergic symptoms.

Avoid eating a lot of spicy food during the pollen season.

They can worsen symptoms and produce similar reactions to allergies, such as runny nose, mouth, and eyes.

Start eating Mediterranean style

Eating fruits, vegetables, healthy grains, legumes, fish, and olive oil—clean, fresh foods—has been shown to aid with a variety of respiratory allergies, including asthma.

Create a long-term, healthy diet to lose extra weight

Numerous studies have definitely shown that obesity may increase the likelihood of asthma episodes in those who already have the condition. Those with this illness might benefit immensely from maintaining a healthy weight.

Use less salt

Regularly cutting back on salt intake can enhance lung function. People should stay away from processed foods as they contain a large amount of salt. When seasoning food, utilize fresh herbs and spices to further cut down on your salt intake.

Kate Kinne, RD, LDN, a dietician at Galter Lifecenter, stated that "Maintaining optimal health is mostly dependent on eating a good diet." For this reason, developing healthy dietary practices can undoubtedly improve how seasonal allergies affect you. No matter how healthy they are now, everyone should aim to consume a range of whole grains, fruits, vegetables, healthy fats, and other simple, unprocessed meals while limiting added salt.

BOOK 16:

Herbs for Women's Fertility and Wellness

For ages, people have turned to herbs as a natural means of boosting fertility and increasing the likelihood of conception. The most often utilized herbs for fertility are maca, red clover, black cohosh, and chasteberry. Herbs have the potential to be an effective tool for supporting general reproductive health when used in conjunction with a nutritious diet and lifestyle choices like regular exercise and stress management practices.

Deciding to become a parent is a significant and occasionally difficult decision. It is crucial to nourish and support your reproductive system if you want to maintain your fertility and become a parent. This is when fertility herbs come in handy.

Herbs can offer you the kind, all-natural support you require.

Herbal treatment for Fertility

Several herbs have been traditionally used to promote fertility in females.

Vitex (Chasteberry)

Vitex, another name for chasteberry, is an herb that has long been used medicinally to increase male and female fertility. A variety of minerals and phytochemicals found in chasteberry fruit extract can assist in regulating hormone levels in the body.

Chasteberry, in particular, may be quite helpful in aiding women who have problems with ovulation and menstruation in getting their progesterone levels back to normal. The chasteberry may also improve male fertility by raising sperm count and motility, according to a number of studies.

Remedy: Consume chasteberry supplements or make a tea from dried chasteberry berries.

Dosage: 400-500 mg of extract or 1-2 cups of tea daily.

Black Cohosh

For its ability to increase fertility, black cohosh is a well-liked plant. This plant contains phytoestrogens and other nutrients, including magnesium and zinc, as well as a number of active chemicals that enhance reproductive health.

According to studies, consuming black cohosh may enhance ovulation and encourage regular menstruation. This herb is often used by women as part of a comprehensive fertility plan, especially when attempting in vitro fertilization or natural conception. Black cohosh is a successful and well-studied natural treatment for boosting fertility and getting the body ready for pregnancy.

Remedy: Consume black cohosh supplements or make a tea from dried black cohosh root.

Dosage: 20-80 mg of extract daily or 1-2 cups of tea daily.

Red Clover

Red clover is a popular and extensively used herb that helps both men and women become more fertile. It is a great option for enhancing reproductive health because of its abundant beneficial components and rich nutrient profile. Men's sperm count and motility may improve thanks to the high magnesium content of red clover. This herb may assist women in controlling their estrogen levels, which may have an impact on both ovulation and the growth of the fetus.

Additionally, red clover is a naturally occurring source of phytoestrogens, which can assist women in regaining balance following periods of hormonal imbalance or instability brought on by specific drugs or therapies.

Remedy: Make a tea from dried red clover flowers or consume red clover supplements.

Dosage: 1-3 cups of tea or 40-160 mg of extract daily.

Evening Primrose Oil

Women have used Evening Primrose oil for millennia as a natural cure for infertility. Omega-3 and omega-6 fatty acids, which are essential for the health of the female reproductive system, are abundant in this plant-based oil. These fatty acids are an excellent medication for women who are having trouble getting pregnant because they may help regulate hormone levels in the body and encourage ovulation.

Evening primrose oil usually doesn't affect the efficacy of regularly prescribed fertility drugs when used in conjunction with them. Once more, nevertheless, it's crucial to consult your physician or the reproductive team.

Remedy: Consume evening primrose oil supplements. Dosage: 500-2000 mg of oil daily.

Maca

Natural plant extract Maca is gaining popularity as a fertility booster. Numerous studies have demonstrated that maca may enhance the reproductive health of both men and women by enhancing the likelihood of conception and a successful pregnancy.

This potent herb creates the perfect environment for pregnancy by balancing hormone levels and improving general health. Maca is a meal that is high in antioxidants and can help shield the body from oxidative stress, which is linked to infertility problems.

Remedy: Consume maca root powder or supplements. Dosage: 1500-3000 mg of extract daily.

Cinnamon

It has long been believed that cinnamon helps with conception. Cinnamaldehyde, a component in cinnamon, has been demonstrated in studies to help regulate hormones and activate the reproductive system.

Additionally, cinnamon has antioxidants that may assist a healthy pregnancy and uterine health by encouraging normal blood flow to the uterus. You may experience excellent reproductive health and increase your chances of conceiving naturally by increasing the amount of cinnamon in your diet.

Remedy: Use cinnamon powder in cooking or make a tea from cinnamon sticks. Dosage: 1-6 grams of powder or 1-2 cups of tea daily.

Ashwagandha

Ashwagandha has been utilized as a reproductive cure for a long time because of its many health advantages. This herbal supplement has potent anti-inflammatory and antioxidant properties, in addition to assisting in hormone regulation and balancing reproductive processes. Ashwagandha is, therefore, a great option for anyone trying to increase their chances of getting pregnant.

Specifically, ashwagandha may help males have higher sperm concentrations, which would boost fertility results. However, in terms of fertility, it might be advantageous for both sexes.

Remedy: Consume ashwagandha root powder or supplements. Dosage: 300-500 mg of extract daily.

Dong Quai

Traditional Chinese medicine has long utilized dong quai, also called Angelica Sinensis, as an infertility remedy. Strong ingredients in this herbal treatment support healthy blood flow and balanced hormone levels in both men and women.

According to studies, dong quai may enhance sperm motility, count, and egg health, all of which can raise the likelihood of pregnancy. Moreover, dong quai may also aid in preventing miscarriage or pre-eclampsia, two pregnancy-related disorders. Dong Quai is a great option for anyone attempting to conceive or seeking natural ways to increase fertility, whether taken as a tablet or steeped into a tea. Remedy: Consume dong quai supplements or make a tea from dried dong quai root. Dosage: 500-1500 mg of extract daily or 1-2 cups of tea daily.

Herbal treatment For Hormone Balance

We frequently encounter moments during the menopausal transition when our hormones become unbalanced, leading to discomfort, hot flashes, nocturnal sweats, exhaustion, fogging of the brain, dietary intolerances, low libido, and insomnia.

The extra stress of modern life, hormone-disrupting chemicals, and environmental contaminants have made this job much more difficult in recent years. Fortunately, several amazing herbs are now accessible to aid with the difficulty.

Black Cohosh

I prefer to use this herbal tincture in my blend of transitional remedies. It helps to maintain estrogen levels. Black cohosh can help by suppressing the luteinizing hormone, which keeps rising when it is trying to find an egg that isn't there, and by acting as a modulator on the estrogen receptor. Estrogen levels can fluctuate as we approach the end of the transition and the actual menopause. In essence, Black Cohosh can be beneficial when there is an excessive swing in estrogen levels. Purchase it from a herbalist, or occasionally discover it in blends for perimenopause. Dosage: 20-80 mg of extract daily or 1-2 ml of tincture three times daily.

Chaste Tree

This is referred to as a hormone regulator since it increases progesterone by suppressing anterior pituitary prolactin. This may help in the latter phases of the shift when there may be greater swings in estrogen, leading to brief periods of temporary estrogen dominance in the body. This may lessen the intensity of hot flashes and nocturnal sweats.

Dosage: 20-40 mg of extract daily or 1-2 ml of tincture daily.

Dong quai

A liver restorative as well as a tonic for women. Supporting the liver and encouraging progesterone production can help prevent hot flashes. Stimulating the pelvic arteries can also help alleviate vaginal dryness.

Dosage: 500-1000 mg of extract daily or 1-2 ml of tincture three times daily.

Ashwagandha

Being a natural adaptogen, this supplement gives your body a wider range of motion to better withstand stress. Supporting the body with a herbal adaptogen is very beneficial since the adrenal glands are not only where we generate hormones that benefit us during and after menopause, but they are also where we regulate stress. An excellent, mild, and helpful herb that reduces inflammation is ashwagandha. (It's not good if your thyroid is overactive.)

Dosage: 300-500 mg of extract daily or 1-2 ml of tincture three times daily.

Passionflower

As progesterone levels drop, sleep might become severely disrupted. This is a lovely plant that promotes sleep by calming the nervous system. During this time, we can also feel a little nervous, and passionflower can help with that.

Dosage: 400-600 mg of extract daily or 1-2 ml of tincture three times daily.

Zizyfus

Zizyfus contains solutions for heart palpitations, sleeplessness, sweats at night, and brain fog. When paired with a passionflower, this kind companion can help you on your path in a variety of ways, making it a synergistic sleep aid.

Dosage: 400-800 mg of extract daily or 1-2 ml of tincture three times daily.

Milk Thistle

Beneficial to the liver. Taking care of your liver might help lessen hot flashes and night sweats since it needs to work harder to process the hormones that fluctuate throughout the later stages of the menopause transition. If your liver is unable to handle these chemicals, your symptoms may get worse. Milk Thistle helps support and process both toxins and hormones since the body prefers to handle contaminants before its own hormones.

Dosage: 200-400 mg of extract daily or 1-2 ml of tincture three times daily.

Herbal treatment for Menopause

Compared to contemporary medicine and therapeutic choices like hormone therapy, herbal therapies for menopause and perimenopause sometimes function differently. Rather than providing controlled relief of presenting symptoms, their natural approach focuses more on preventing and lessening the severity of symptoms.

For the best outcome for a patient, many doctors nowadays would advise a combined therapy approach that makes use of both more conventional medicines and the most recent advancements in medical science.

Black Cohosh

Uses: Alleviates hot flashes, night sweats, and mood swings.

Dosage: 20-80 mg of extract daily or 1-2 ml of tincture three times daily.

Chaste Tree

Uses: Regulates hormones by inhibiting prolactin, increasing progesterone, and reducing menopausal symptoms such as hot flashes and night sweats.

Dosage: 20-40 mg of extract daily or 1-2 ml of tincture daily.

Dong Quai

Uses: Acts as a female tonic and liver restorative, supports the production of progesterone, alleviates hot flashes, and reduces vaginal dryness.

Dosage: 500-1000 mg of extract daily or 1-2 ml of tincture three times daily.

Ashwagandha

Uses: Herbal adaptogen that supports adrenal health, manages stress and has anti- inflammatory properties.

Dosage: 300-500 mg of extract daily or 1-2 ml of tincture three times daily.

Red Clover

Uses: Contains phytoestrogens that help reduce hot flashes and improve bone health. Dosage: 40-80 mg of extract daily or 2-4 grams of dried flowers steeped in tea.

Evening Primrose Oil

Uses: Provides relief from hot flashes, night sweats, and mood swings. Dosage: 500-1000 mg of oil daily in divided doses.

Maca

Uses: Balances hormones, boosts energy levels, and reduces menopausal symptoms. Dosage: 1-3 grams of powder daily or 500-1000 mg of extract daily.

Sage

Uses: Reduces hot flashes and excessive sweating.

Dosage: 300-600 mg of extract daily or 1-2 grams of dried leaves steeped in tea.

Licorice Root

Uses: Mimics estrogen, helping to balance hormones and reduce hot flashes. Dosage: 1-2 grams of dried root steeped in tea or 250-500 mg of extract daily.

St. John's Wort

Uses: Improves mood, reduces anxiety, and alleviates symptoms of mild depression during menopause.

Dosage: 300-600 mg of extract three times daily.

Herbal treatment for Menstrual Disorders

Dysmenorrhea, or painful period, is characterized by pains in the thighs, back, and lower abdomen. Days before your menstrual cycle starts, you may have menstrual cramps. Prostaglandins are inflammatory chemicals that resemble hormones and induce the uterus to contract and shed its lining. This is the bleeding of your menstruation. Herbal teas can help reduce inflammation and balance hormones, which will lessen period-related pains like headaches, cramps, and mood changes. Here are some fantastic herbs that are frequently used as a natural remedy to support a healthy menstrual cycle and aid with PMS symptoms.

Chasteberry

Native to western Asia and the Mediterranean, chaste berries have been used since ancient times. Recent research has found that these berries have hormonal qualities that balance hormones. It is believed that chaste berries improve hormonal issues by acting on the pituitary gland and increasing progesterone levels. Additionally, by doing these steps, PMS symptoms, including mood swings, breast discomfort, and regular menstruation, are relieved.

Raspberry Leaf

Although raspberries are often thought of for their delicious, fruity flavor, raspberry leaf tea has long been utilized as a uterine toning agent. The raspberry leaf is frequently used to reduce PMS symptoms, ease menstrual pain, and manage heavy monthly bleeding. You can get much-needed relief throughout your cycle by sipping a hot cup of raspberry leaf tea.

Chamomile

Chamomile is frequently utilized for its calming and relaxing properties. These activities assist in reducing anxiety. The Romans were among the first to utilize chamomile to relieve menstrual pains. These days, chamomile is an excellent option for PMS alleviation.

Fennel

Fennel is frequently used as a digestive aid to lessen gas and bloating. Period pain can also be relieved with fennel. Fennel helps lessen unpredictable menstruation cycles and discomfort when taken over several months. Fennel is a need if you want to relieve PMS symptoms.

Wild Yam

Period pain and other menopausal symptoms are frequently relieved with wild yam. This root has hormonal, anti-inflammatory, and pain-relieving properties. Among the plants that lower inflammation is wild yam. Period cramps can be lessened with these practices.

Herbal treatment for Pregnancy

Anxiety, back discomfort, nausea, and morning sickness are common side effects of pregnancy. Even while it's not always a good idea to use medication, you might want to think about trying some natural therapies at home, such as pregnancy-safe herbal teas. Herbal medicines are generally seen as a healthy and safe alternative, but using them when pregnant calls for particular caution. Let's examine herbs during pregnancy: What is and is not safe.

When used sparingly, the following herbs are thought to be safe during pregnancy:

Ginger

Almost every Indian kitchen has a special spot for this fragrant, spicy plant. While some pregnant women find that ginger ale helps ease nausea, most pregnant women prefer ginger tea.

Peppermint

When you're pregnant, peppermint, one of the most popular herbs, has multiple uses. Mint helps with nausea and flatulence, but too much of it is not suggested. It can be added to lemonade, used as pregnancy teas, or made into chutney.

Eucalyptus

If you have a cold while pregnant, taking a tablet might not be the best course of action. It can be applied as a sinus-relieving essential oil.

Cranberry

Cranberry juice is a simple and safe way to avoid urinary tract infections, or UTIs, which are frequent during pregnancy. Prefer homemade cranberry juice that is produced fresh and has less sugar.

Chamomile

One of the discomforts that pregnancy may bring about for you is disturbed sleep. Chamomile tea is tasty and calming; you can have it once or twice a day. It is well- known for promoting restful sleep and for its soothing scent.

Red Raspberry Leaf

Red raspberry leaf may help to support a healthy pregnancy, according to studies. It helps prepare you for a simple birth and tones the uterus. It is also thought to hasten labor, which lowers the need for interventions and/or birth-related problems.

While using herbs during pregnancy is a personal decision, you should be well- informed on the different kinds of herbs, their uses (tea, tonic, capsule, etc.), and their parts (root, leaf, etc.) to ensure the best possible outcome for you and your unborn child. Food or tonic herbs are frequently those regarded as safe to use during pregnancy. Usually, you can find these as tablets, tea, or infusions.

Herbal treatment for Postpartum

The quantity of advice you may receive during your pregnancy might be overwhelming, particularly if you don't ask for it! There's a lot of enthusiasm, and the pregnant mother receives a lot of advice, attention, and pampering. However, most new parents have to wing it when it comes to postpartum healing.

When I think of the movie Birdbox, I usually see Sandra Bullock feeling her way to safety while blindfolded and accompanied by her kids through dangerous woods while loud music plays.

In terms of medicine, the advice is frequently to "take an NSAID like Tylenol and ibuprofen for pain" and nothing more.

In general, there are more choices. Natural treatments can help with the emotional changes that happen during the postpartum period, in addition to supporting physical resilience and healing.

Skullcap

I always associate wearing a skullcap with emerging from one's head (see what I did there, head, skull, eh eh?) For people dealing with worry, stress-related restlessness, and insomnia—which might be considered the epitome of the postpartum experience—skullcap is an excellent herb for boosting mood. If a parent is having headaches, difficulty falling or staying asleep, or minor postpartum mood issues, skullcap should be seriously explored.

Ashwagandha

A helpful herb for anyone recuperating from stress is ashwagandha. It is a friend of the overburdened and overworked. It functions as a general tonic for the body, supporting hormone and cortisol homeostasis. It helps the body readjust following sleep pattern disruptions caused by overstressed adrenal glands. It specifically targets the adrenal glands. When combined with Shatavari root, it is extremely beneficial for nursing mothers.

Holy Basil

In a cup, holy basil feels like a comfortable old friend. In terms of medicine, it functions as an adaptogen that helps balance out after stress. It can be used for an extended period of time, acting as a tonic for the body to boost energy, increase resilience against chronic stress, and enhance mood in cases of moderate postpartum depression.

Nettle

An incredible herb to use before, during, and after pregnancy is nettle. After birth, it fortifies the kidneys and adrenal glands. Our bodies are flooded with hormones after giving birth. The liver and kidneys process and eliminate hormones from the body; if these organs are functioning slowly, the excess hormones may overwhelm them, resulting in noticeable mood swings, acne, and an overall sense of exhaustion.

Moringa

As a dietary supplement, tonic, astringent, antioxidant, anti-inflammatory, and immune system booster, I recommend moringa leaves to newlyweds. The body is exhausted after giving birth and needs nourishment to repair itself. Iron, calcium, and phosphorus are abundant in moringa, a complete protein. It is also a fantastic breastfeeding assistance.

Herbal treatment for Urinary Tract Health

Bacteria are typically the cause of UTIs. Antibiotics could be necessary in certain situations to eradicate the infection. However, this isn't always required. Herbal medicines that target the elimination of dangerous germs from your system can also be used at home.

Numerous herbs also include antibacterial qualities, which aid in eliminating the microorganisms causing your illness.

Uva ursi

For generations, uva ursi, also referred to as bearberry, has been utilized as a herbal remedy for utis. It originates from a tiny, native American evergreen shrub and is still widely used as a treatment for kidney stones and utis.

As a naturally occurring diuretic, uva ursi promotes increased urine production, which aids in the removal of dangerous microorganisms from our bodies.

In addition to its antibacterial qualities, uva ursi contains an antiseptic and analgesic chemical called arbutin.

Parsley

The use of parsley tea as a home treatment for utis is also common. Parsley, which is likely most recognized for its usage as a culinary garnish, is a powerhouse of antioxidants and antibacterial qualities that inhibit the growth of bacteria like Escherichia coli, one of the most prevalent causes of utis.

Similar to uva ursi, parsley is a mild diuretic and can aid in clearing your urinary tract of bacteria that cause UTIs.

Juniper berry

The small, dark berries of the juniper bush have long been utilized as a home cure for kidney problems and utis, in addition to being used in gin production.

Because juniper is a diuretic, it causes our bodies to secrete more pee. This not only aids in maintaining fluid balance but also helps our bodies eliminate pathogenic germs.

In addition, these berries contain antimicrobial essential oils that stop the formation of utis-causing bacteria.

Cranberry

Many individuals use cranberries as a natural cure for utis infections since they are arguably the most well-known.

In contrast to several other herbs on our list, cranberries don't seem to work as a bacteria-killing agent to prevent utis. Rather, the substances present in these tiny red berries aid in preventing bacteria from sticking to the urinary tract's walls.

Consequently, this facilitates our bodies' ability to eliminate infections through urine. For optimal results, you might want to combine cranberries with some of the diuretic herbs on our list.

Acerola

Though it's not a true cherry, the fruit of the acerola tree has a striking resemblance to a cherry. This fruit, which is native to the Americas, has a lot of nutrients, especially vitamin C.

Because of its high vitamin C content, acerola is particularly beneficial for people who frequently get utis. It increases the acidity of your urine, which inhibits the growth of bacteria in your urinary system.

Additionally, vitamin C strengthens your immune system, which makes it easier for your body to fend against infections.

Goldenseal

Goldenseal is another plant that is frequently used to treat uTIs. This herb, which is native to North America, contains antibacterial and anti-inflammatory qualities that aid in the battle against bacteria that might cause utis.

Berberine, a substance found in goldenseal, is mostly responsible for the herb's anti- utis properties. It is easier to get rid of bacteria before they produce an illness because berberine makes it more difficult for them to adhere to the walls of the urinary system.

BOOK 17:

Herbal Healing for Children

Children are unique beings with developing bodies that are incredibly sensitive and attentive. They have a lot of energy and are kind and understanding. The source of our lives' brightness. Since they are human, they occasionally become ill, just like humans. When this occurs, it's critical to keep in mind that their small bodies require a delicate healing process. It's normal to desire to call the doctor as soon as possible in many situations. We desire for our little ones to recover as quickly as possible. Seeing your child struggle with a cough that keeps them awake at night or breathing difficulties due to congestion is really upsetting. A doctor usually prescribes a prescription treatment, an over-the-counter medication, or advises rest and plenty of fluids. Medicinal herbs are a great substitute for other pharmaceuticals that frequently include questionable components and have adverse effects. A more holistic doctor may advise using them.

Plants with components and compounds that aid in healing in a variety of ways are known as medicinal herbs. This kind of use of plants dates back at least 60,000 years. The use of plants as medicine has long existed in every culture on Earth. A lot of that information has been forgotten or lost over time. Luckily for us, we have access to an abundance of knowledge nowadays. This facilitates the process of determining which plants to utilize and why. The results of ongoing scientific research confirm what people have long known—that medicinal plants are effective. Not all herbs are suitable for youngsters, though, as I have indicated, because some are delicate and require a more delicate approach. However, a number of them—some referred to as "children's herbs"—do well with kids, are risk-free, and have no negative side effects. Consequently, children can use safe and efficient herbal medicines!

First, let's talk about immune-boosting herbs.

You can give your child these herbs as soon as they show symptoms of illness. These can also be used as a prophylactic measure to maintain robust and activated immune systems for a set period of time (for example, the entire winter season) or after your child has been exposed to an infection. Astragalus, Elderberry, and Echinacea have all received a lot of attention recently. This is due to scientific studies demonstrating that consuming these extracts can help reduce the length of time that colds and the flu last. In addition to being safe for kids, all three of these plants include antiviral, anti-inflammatory, and antiseptic properties that work to strengthen the immune system.

Although strengthening the immune system is beneficial, more herbs are frequently required for more specialized conditions, such as a child's cough. Numerous herbs are beneficial for maintaining a healthy respiratory system. But how can you choose which one to use? Well, coughs usually come in a variety of forms. Let's talk about a wet cough and a dry cough to keep things easy. Herbal demulcents are soothing and moisturizing remedies for dry cough. Marshmallow is my go-to child-soothing agent. Herbs that reduce spasms are also helpful in this situation, as they can aid in falling asleep and lessen persistent coughing. This includes Mullein, Red Clover, and Thyme. Using expectorants for a wet cough can assist in moving mucus out of the lungs and up, which will make coughing more productive. Marshmallow, mullein, thyme, and hornehound are excellent expectorants for children. Wild Cherry Bark is also a great option if your child has a sore throat.

My top three "multi-purpose" herbs for kids are probably chamomile, catnip, and lemon balm. I suggest keeping some or all of these herbs on hand so you can create tea for your family and child. They're all really tasty as well! Both catnip and lemon balm have nervine, antiviral, antibacterial, and antifungal properties. They aid in boosting the immune system and calming the mind, easing tension, anxiety, and restlessness. Since they belong to the mint family, they are also soothing to the digestive system and excellent for upset stomachs and colic. Despite being in a distinct family, chamomile possesses comparable qualities. It is a mild sedative that is mostly used to support sleep, soothe upset stomachs, and lessen the symptoms of ADHD. (As chamomile belongs to the same family as ragweed, avoid using it if your child develops an allergy to it.)

Other herbs I love for kids (and for mamas & papas):

Rich in vitamins and minerals, nettle, red clover, and red raspberry leaf are extremely nourishing herbs. These taste well with tea. My son and I often drink a "nourishing" combination that I brew in the morning.

Tulsi, often known as holy basil, is another fantastic herb with many uses. It helps the neurological system, boosts immunity, enhances memory, and does a tonne of other things. In India, this plant is cultivated in practically every home and is revered as a goddess!

Here are a few more: peppermint, elderflower, lavender, and calendula.

You now own an extensive list of possible solutions to assist your child in the future. But which ones should you use and how do you take them? Herbal medicine can be applied in a variety of ways, depending on the patient. Herbs can be applied topically, consumed as tinctures, made into teas, and given as herbal baths. Though glycerites, which are prepared with vegetable glycerin, are occasionally referred to as tinctures, tinctures are typically extracts of alcohol. Glycerin is used in the majority of tinctures sold to children because it is sweeter and easier for kids to take. Take it slow when using herbs at first. Find what suits your family's needs. When your child is unwell, is it easier to give them a dropperful of tincture and maybe a cup or two of tea, or is your child eager to drink many cups of tea?

I advise always carrying one tincture for respiratory health and one for immune strengthening (containing either Echinacea or Astragalus). I also strongly suggest making or purchasing elderberry syrup if you can. I switch between the immune-boosting tincture and the elderberry syrup when my child is unwell. In addition, I enjoy keeping a combination of herbal teas for immunity and respiratory health, as well as some delicious teas for kids, like chamomile and lemon balm. I have to admit that I adore herbal chest rubs as well. I've been giving my child herbal chest rubs every night to help with breathing while he sleeps because they work so well for regular use and are especially effective when he has a cough. And last, since most kids enjoy taking baths, herbal steams, and baths are great ways to introduce other herbs to youngsters! You may use any herbs for this, but my favorites are calendula, lemon balm, chamomile, lavender, and thyme. Depending on the circumstance, combinations of herbs or single herbs can be employed successfully.

Hopefully, having this knowledge will enable you to support your family's holistic health journey. Please be aware that the provided information is not meant to be a substitute for or reflect the advise of a doctor or other medical expert. Always get medical advice first, as certain herbs might not be suitable for you in particular. I always advise you to do additional research so that you can use medicinal herbs with your family with confidence and a sense of empowerment from having the most knowledge.

Digestive Issues

Children often experience digestive discomfort, including indigestion, bloating, and constipation. Several herbs can help soothe their tummies:

Ginger:

Uses: Relieves nausea, indigestion, and gas.

Dosage: For children over 2 years, 1-2 grams of fresh ginger steeped in hot water can be given as tea.

Chamomile:

Uses: Soothes upset stomachs, reduces gas, and alleviates colic.

Dosage: 1-2 teaspoons of dried chamomile flowers steeped in a cup of hot water. Safe for infants in small amounts.

Peppermint:

Uses: Eases stomach cramps and indigestion.

Dosage: 1 teaspoon of dried peppermint leaves steeped in hot water for children over 2 years old.

Immune Support

Strengthening the immune system is crucial for children, especially during cold and flu season. These herbs can help boost their immunity:

Elderberry:

Uses: Prevents and treats colds and flu.

Dosage: Elderberry syrup, 1 teaspoon daily for children over 1 year old.

Echinacea:

Uses: Enhances immune function and helps fight infections.

Dosage: Echinacea tincture, 5-10 drops diluted in water, for children over 2 years old.

Astragalus:

Uses: Boosts immune function and helps prevent illness.

Dosage: Astragalus root tea, 1 cup daily for children over 2 years old.

Skin Conditions

From eczema to minor cuts and scrapes, children's skin can benefit from the healing properties of certain herbs:

Calendula:

Uses: Treats eczema, rashes, and minor wounds.

Dosage: Apply calendula cream or ointment topically as needed.

Aloe Vera:

Uses: Soothes burns, rashes, and insect bites.

Dosage: Apply fresh aloe vera gel directly to the affected area.

Lavender:

Uses: Calms irritated skin and promotes healing.

Dosage: Dilute lavender essential oil in a carrier oil and apply it to the skin.

Cognitive Development

Supporting cognitive development and mental clarity can be achieved with these gentle herbs:

Ginkgo Biloba:

Uses: Enhances memory and cognitive function.

Dosage: For children over 5 years old, 30-60 mg of standardized extract daily.

Lemon Balm:

Uses: Calms the mind and improves concentration.

Dosage: Lemon balm tea, 1-2 cups daily for children over 2 years old.

Brahmi:

Uses: Supports brain function and learning.

Dosage: For children over 5 years old, 300-500 mg of standardized extract daily.

Allergies

Herbal remedies can provide relief from common allergy symptoms such as sneezing and itchy eyes:

Nettle:

Uses: Reduces allergy symptoms like sneezing and itching.

Dosage: Nettle leaf tea, 1-2 cups daily for children over 5 years old.

Butterbur:

Uses: Alleviates hay fever symptoms.

Dosage: For children over 6 years old, 50-75 mg of standardized extract twice daily.

Quercetin:

Uses: Acts as a natural antihistamine.

Dosage: For children over 5 years old, 100-200 mg daily.

Respiratory Health

Maintaining respiratory health is essential, especially during the cold season. The following herbs can help:

Thyme (Thymus vulgaris):

Uses: Eases coughs and clears congestion.

Dosage: Thyme tea, 1-2 cups daily for children over 2 years old.

Marshmallow Root (Althaea officinalis):

Uses: Soothes sore throats and alleviates coughs.

Dosage: Marshmallow root tea, 1-2 cups daily for children over 2 years old.

Mullein (Verbascum thapsus):

Uses: Supports lung health and clears mucus.

Dosage: Mullein tea, 1-2 cups daily for children over 5 years old.

Herbal treatments provide a safe, all-natural means of promoting children's health in a variety of ailments. To guarantee safety and appropriate dosage, it is imperative to speak with a pediatric herbalist or healthcare professional before introducing any new herb. These herbal medicines might be useful instruments for promoting your child's health and wellbeing if used under the proper supervision.

BOOK 18:

Growing and Sourcing Your Own

Herbs

I'm asked this question all the time: "Where do you obtain all your herbs? Are these all that you grow yourself? I need MANY more herbs than I could ever grow myself because I make herbal medicine for more people than just myself, and not all of the herbs I use in my practice are even climate-appropriate. I believe I should speak up in favor of ethical herb sourcing, given the recent surge in interest in wildcrafting, cultivating one's own herbs, and producing herbal medicine.

Cultivate

My first choice when it comes to obtaining herbs is to grow my own. It not only saves the money and the carbon footprint associated with ordering herbs online and having them transported to you, but it also allows me to get to know the plant better. Growing your own herbs, whether from seed or seedling, encourages you to learn about the requirements of the plant for light, water, companion plants, when and if pruning is necessary, pests and diseases it is susceptible to, growth habits throughout its life cycle, and the most effective way to propagate it.

Your ability to identify plants is further enhanced by keeping an eye on them during all phases of their life, from growth to death. What's the appearance of calendula seeds? Is there a scent difference between comfrey and elecampane roots? To avoid pulling weeds, can you identify the young self-healing leaves among the others? Given that the marshmallow's name includes the word "marsh," should you move it to a wetter location? You have the most intimate knowledge of herbs when you cultivate and harvest them yourself. Although I understand that not everyone has the space to do this outside, you may cultivate a relationship with plants, even with only a pot of tulsi on your windowsill or a container garden on your patio or balcony.

Asking friends and neighbors if they have what you need is an additional option. I've frequently found just what I need by posting about herbs in local Facebook groups. Perhaps there aren't many unusual herbs like this one in your area, but your neighbor may have a huge rosemary shrub that they're unsure how to use. Alternatively, you may ask a buddy who has a larger garden than you to grow some produce for you. This would also make a great foundation for a cooperative medicinal herb garden!

Wildcraft

"Can I wildcraft this?" is the next thing I ask myself if I am unable to produce the plant myself. When I initially heard the term "wildcrafting," I immediately thought of an adventurous, well-prepared hiker carrying a knife into the forest. It doesn't need to be this difficult. With my collecting apron as my only instrument, I can gather honeysuckle wild in my own backyard while wearing only my bare feet. That's about all the fancy gear I need; on occasion, I scout out a wildcrafting area while driving, tossing some baskets and my favorite pair of Felcos in the car. On other occasions, I would just toss some reishi mushrooms into my pocket while taking a stroll through the woods. That's wildcrafting; it's that easy.

The process of wildcrafting plants involves various factors. Determine whether the area is sufficiently clean to harvest first. Never pick plants from the side of a busy road or from a farmer's field adjacent to one that uses herbicides and pesticides. If you notice those signs with the seed business and seed lot numbers along the field's edge, you can be sure this is what it is. The farmer most likely bought his seeds from a large agricultural business like Dow or Monsanto, which implies the plants are round-up ready and genetically modified. Municipalities frequently spray herbicides beside roadsides. Ask yourself, "Do I need permission to wildcraft here?" after that. It's usually a good practice to get permission from landowners before harvesting, even if what you are chasing is "weeds" to them. It's also crucial to have the consent of the plants you plan to use to manufacture medication. The basic norm is to take only what you need or one-third of what is there, whichever is less, if you feel comfortable on the property. Above all, it's critical to ascertain whether the plant you wish to work with is endangered, threatened, or sacred to a culture other than your own. An excellent source of information about plants that run the risk of being overharvested is the United Plant Savers website, which also provides a list of analogs for at-risk herbs. I wildcraft a lot of local herbs in my area, such as yarrow, violet, and goldenrod. They're not in danger; I can find them easily, and they grow so abundantly in the wild that I don't need to take up valuable garden space to grow them.

Finding invasive plants to harvest for medicinal purposes is even better because it relieves some of the ecosystem's strain by eliminating some of the non-native species. When referring to plants, I really don't even want to use the term "invasive" because it seems like such a bad thing. Additionally, native plants like ground ivy that just have an aggressive growth habit are sometimes referred to as "invasive" by people. Many of them naturalized after escaping cultivation and arriving here as ornamentals. However, not all of them are bad; some of them are getting along well with their new companions. Non-native plants that I frequently collect include mimosa, purple loosestrife, and Japanese honeysuckle. In my region of the planet, there are a lot of non-native plants that are highly beneficial for usage as food and medicine. Some allies I can find nearby if I need them include purple loosestrife, autumn olive, Japanese barberry (an analog of goldenseal), and garlic mustard.

Purchase

If I am unable to produce or wildcraft the necessary herbs, I will either purchase them in bulk online, visit my neighborhood herb store, or try to find a grower whose ethics coincide with mine. In order to grow plants like echinacea root, ashwagandha, blue vervain, and calendula that I don't have room for in my partly shaded woodland garden, I've even collaborated with my neighborhood CSA farmer.

There are two things you can do when buying herbs. Purchasing in large quantities or in tiny amounts. Which is superior?

For myself, I engage in both. I purchase a tiny quantity of a herb while I'm testing it out for the first time. I purchase a tiny quantity of unusual herbs when using them in particular remedies. I purchase common herbs in bulk if I intend to use them in a variety of ways. I purchase in bulk if I'm preparing a big meal for friends and family. This is my method.

You may get herbs by the ounce at a lot of the nearby health food stores. I'm not referring to ready-made tinctures, tea packages, or even herbal supplements. I'm referring to dried, loose herbs that you can buy and use whatever you please. This is usually the best approach to buying herbs because you can determine how much you need, which is ideal if you just need a tiny amount or are just testing it out.

Nonetheless, purchasing in bulk is frequently preferable if you want to stock up on herbs or if you are preparing a large quantity of something.

Mountain Rose Herbs

The biggest assortment of herbs that I am aware of may be found at Mountain Rose Herbs, another fantastic online herbal retailer. I enjoy looking around their website! In addition to herbs, they provide a wide range of supplies needed to create a variety of herbal, domestic, and skin care cures. The majority of their herbs are wild-crafted or certified organic, and they are available in 4 oz, 8 oz, or 1-pound bags for small batch and bulk purchases.

Starwest Botanicals and Frontier Herbs

Bulk quantities of natural and organic herbs are available from Starwest Botanicals and Frontier

Herbs. I frequently buy bulk herbs from these two suppliers on Amazon; they often have sizes of 8 oz and 1 pound.

How To Source Quality Herbs

When high-quality herbs aren't used, it can be one of the reasons herbal remedies don't work and why beginners give up on them altogether. Like most things in life, quality counts, and you will typically have to spend more for higher-quality goods.

Now, try not to worry. Even while you might spend a little more on high-quality herbs than a lower-quality variety, you'll still finish up ahead financially when you use herbs yourself rather than purchasing readymade items or visiting a doctor.

How then do you find high-quality herbs? When searching for high-quality herbs, bear the following four points in mind.

Freshness

An herb's freshness is important. This is why the majority of consumers who begin purchasing smaller amounts of spices from spice firms never return to using the bottled spices that are displayed on the shelves of their local grocery stores. How long have those herbs been in those bottles and on the shelf, do you know? I know the spices I buy from my neighborhood health food store taste far better than mine, but I don't!

Dates on the herbs that local and internet sellers buy and sell are typically monitored. This aids in their product rotation since they may replace stale herbs with fresher ones. Since such herbs aren't in season and can't be purchased from the herb growers they deal with, many herb wholesalers will actually run out of stock of some herbs at different periods of the year.

Thus, how can one determine whether a herb is fresh?

Ask first! The majority of store owners are glad to provide you with this information.

Look at the herb next. Is it bright and vibrant, or is it faded and dull? Are you unsure about the intended appearance? Before you buy, do some online research. You can tell a fresher herb from an old one by knowing what a high-quality herb looks like.

You can also take a whiff of the herb. Of course, this is limited to nearby herb stores, but in most cases, you can open the herbal container and smell it. If it has an herbal scent, it's probably still fresh enough to use and has some therapeutic value.

And lastly, it tastes good. The plant is probably fresh if it has a lot of flavors—be it sweet, salty, pungent, spicy, or bitter.

Herb labels

You'll frequently see herbs labeled as "natural," "organic," and "wild-crafted" when looking for herbs. Here are the definitions of each of those terms along with my personal favourite.

Natural

A "natural" herb's label doesn't tell you much. An herb is naturally occurring—after all, it's a plant! To improve the appearance of their product, companies will occasionally label herbs as "natural" or "grown without chemicals," but in my opinion, this is insufficient. When it comes time to use my herbs, I want to know that they are chemical-free, picked during prime seasons, and then dried and stored properly to keep them as fresh as possible.

Granted, not every herb firm sells organic or wild-crafted herbs, which isn't always a bad thing, but in this case, doing your homework and having faith in the company is important. More on that will be covered below.

Organic

Herbs that bear the labels "organic" or "certified organic" are grown without the use of dangerous, synthetic chemicals and are not handled in any way after harvest. Although a product isn't always of good quality just because it is labeled as "organic," this is certainly one of the better selections you can find to buy. High quality involves more than just avoiding chemicals. Once more, harvesting, processing, and storage are all relevant.

The majority of businesses that sell herbs that have been "certified organic" will have an organic seal or label indicating where they obtained their certifications on their product or website. Because they are honest with their facts, this is also an excellent sign of a trustworthy organization.

I can already see someone asking me if it truly makes a difference to purchase "certified organic" herbs. Yes and no, respectively, would be my response to that query. Purchasing herbs with labels declaring they are organic gives you a sense of quality, assurance, and trust. But what about tiny enterprises or local herb growers who cannot afford to obtain that official label? They might still provide premium organic herbs; they just lack a label or certificate to support that claim. Once more, this is a matter of personal preference and necessitates learning more about herbs from companies who do not sell "certified organic" goods. Small companies that seem to want your business are usually honest about how they procure, prepare, and store herbs.

Wildcrafted

Herbs collected from the wild can be just as excellent as organic ones, if not better. When it comes to their therapeutic properties, wild-crafted herbs are often of a higher grade than many herbs grown on farms. These are plants that have been harvested directly from their natural habitat.

The market for ginseng is one place where this is evident. Compared to produced ginseng roots, wild ginseng roots grow differently and are smaller. Just by examining the root, buyers may determine whether ginseng is wild or cultivated, and wild "sang" is thus more expensive to buy and sell than cultivated ginseng.

Don't get me wrong; there are some really excellent herbs grown on farms. Research and confidence in the vendor are crucial in this situation as well.

You must be aware of each company's policies regarding wildcrafting. There are rules, and if you don't make sure your herbs are sustainably wildcrafted, they can become extinct, and you won't be able to obtain them. Because farm-raised herbs aren't overharvested, this is one way that they can be superior to wild-crafted herbs.

Harvesting practices

Harvesting methods provide another means of assessing an herb's quality.

Why then are harvesting practices important? To maintain the maximum amount of their medicinal qualities, some plants need to be gathered and prepared in a specific method. This can include the best times to harvest (buds vs. open flowers, spring or fall harvesting, first-year vs. second-year plants, etc.); how to store freshly harvested plants before drying (sun vs. shade); how to dry the plant (method, temperature, etc.); and how to handle and store the dried plant thereafter (including shipping).

If you question a corporation, ideally, they will know how their farmers gather herbs. If they don't, it could be an indication that the business doesn't place a high value on herbal quality.

Storage

When searching for high-quality herbs, the way the herb is stored should be your final consideration. Herbs are best kept in an airtight, cool, dark storage environment.

Herbs are typically kept in glass jars at local markets, which reduces oxygen exposure and keeps the herb free of dust and insects. Most online retailers will package herbs in plastic bags for delivery. Since every company operates differently, you are welcome to inquire about the method used to store these herbs prior to their being put in bags.

Regarding quality, the temperature at which the herb is stored also counts. Because heat above 100 degrees Fahrenheit harms the components of plants, they should not be stored in any area that is hotter than that.

As with high temperatures and oxygen, light exposure also degrades the qualities of herbs, so it's best to avoid it. Herbs are stored well in dark bottles, paper-covered glass jars or tins, or paper bags that block light.

How to grow an Herb Garden

Enjoying the beauty and scent of fresh herbs while expanding your culinary and medicinal toolset is a rewarding and useful approach to growing an herb garden. This guide will walk you through every step of growing a successful herb garden, regardless of your level of gardening experience.

Planning Your Herb Garden

Choose Your Location:

Sunlight: Most herbs require at least 6-8 hours of direct sunlight each day. Choose a sunny spot in your garden or on a windowsill if you're growing indoors.

Soil: Herbs prefer well-drained soil. If your soil is heavy clay or sandy, consider amending it with organic matter like compost to improve drainage and fertility.

Space: Consider the size and spread of your herbs. Some, like mint, can spread aggressively, so it's important to plan for adequate space or use containers.

Select Your Herbs:

Culinary Herbs: Basil, rosemary, thyme, oregano, chives, parsley, mint, and cilantro are popular choices.

Medicinal Herbs: Echinacea, chamomile, lavender, and calendula are beneficial for home remedies.

Companion Planting: Some herbs can deter pests and enhance the growth of neighboring plants. For example, basil can repel aphids and improve the flavor of tomatoes.

Preparing the Soil

Test Your Soil:

pH Level: Herbs generally prefer a slightly acidic to neutral pH (6.0-7.0). Test your soil using a pH test kit and amend it if necessary.

Nutrients: Incorporate organic matter, such as compost or aged manure, to provide essential nutrients and improve soil structure.

Prepare the Bed:

Weeding: Clear the area of weeds and debris.

Tilling: Loosen the soil to a depth of about 12 inches (30 cm) to promote root growth and improve drainage.

Planting Your Herbs

Starting from Seeds:

Indoor Seedlings: Start seeds indoors 6-8 weeks before the last expected frost date. Use seed trays or pots with a light, well-draining seed starting mix.

Direct Sowing: Some herbs, like cilantro and dill, can be sown directly into the garden once the soil has warmed.

Transplanting Seedlings:

Hardening Off: Gradually acclimate indoor seedlings to outdoor conditions over a week.

Planting: Dig holes slightly larger than the root ball of each seedling. Space the plants according to their mature size and growth habits.

Container Gardening:

Choosing Containers: Select containers with drainage holes. Terra cotta pots are a good choice as they allow air circulation to the roots.

Potting Mix: Use a high-quality potting mix designed for container gardening.

Caring for Your Herb Garden

Watering:

Frequency: Water regularly, but avoid overwatering. Most herbs prefer slightly dry conditions over being waterlogged.

Method: Water the base of the plants to prevent fungal diseases.

Mulching:

Benefits: Mulch helps retain soil moisture, suppress weeds, and regulate soil temperature.

Materials: Use organic mulch like straw, shredded leaves, or compost.

Fertilizing:

Type: Use a balanced, organic fertilizer or compost.

Frequency: Herbs generally don't need heavy fertilizing. Once or twice a season is usually sufficient.

Pruning and Harvesting:

Pruning: Regularly pinch back the growing tips to encourage bushier growth and prevent flowering, which can make herbs bitter.

Harvesting: Harvest herbs in the morning after the dew has dried but before the heat of the day. Use sharp scissors or pruning shears to cut the stems.

Dealing with Pests and Diseases

Common Pests:

Aphids: Spray with a mixture of water and mild soap.

Spider Mites: Increase humidity around the plants and use insecticidal soap. Slugs and Snails: Use barriers like crushed eggshells or diatomaceous earth.

Common Diseases:

Powdery Mildew: Ensure good air circulation and avoid overhead watering. Root Rot: Avoid waterlogged soil by ensuring proper drainage.

Winterizing Your Herb Garden

Bringing Indoors:

Pots: Move potted herbs indoors before the first frost. Light: Place them in a sunny window or use grow lights.

Outdoor Protection:

Mulch: Apply a thick layer of mulch around the base of perennial herbs to protect the roots from freezing temperatures.

Cover: Use cloches or row covers to protect herbs from frost.

Enjoying and Using Your Herbs

Culinary Uses:

Fresh: Use fresh herbs to enhance the flavor of your dishes.

Drying: Hang herbs in a cool, dry place or use a dehydrator to preserve them.

Medicinal Uses:

Teas: Brew herbs like chamomile and peppermint for soothing teas.

Salves and Oils: Infuse herbs like calendula and lavender in oils for skin care remedies.

Growing an herb garden is a delightful and rewarding endeavor that can provide fresh, flavorful, and medicinal herbs throughout the year. By following these steps and processes, you can cultivate a thriving herb garden that brings both beauty and utility to your home.

BOOK 19:

Nutritious Recipes and Meal Plans

Welcome to " Nutritious Recipes and Meal Plans" a gastronomic adventure that blends delectable recipes created to nourish your body and enhance well-being with the knowledge of holistic nutrition. The principles of Dr. Barbara O'Neill, a well-known proponent of natural health and diet, served as the inspiration for this cookbook.

Embracing nutrient-dense foods

In this cookbook, there are many recipes that highlight nutrient-dense foods like fresh fruits, vegetables, whole grains, nuts, seeds, and legumes. These foods are high in fiber, antioxidants, vitamins, and minerals—all of which are necessary for maintaining optimum health and vitality.

Principles of holistic nutrition

This cookbook is based on the holistic nutrition approach of Dr. Barbara O'Neill. Her tenets highlight:

Plant-based emphasis: dishes that highlight the variety of plant-based foods that are high in nutrients and well-known for their therapeutic qualities.

Whole and natural: this approach promotes the use of unprocessed, whole ingredients to maintain their nutritional value and improve their health-promoting attributes.

Alkaline and balanced: encouraging a diet that is both balanced and supports the body's alkaline balance, which is thought to lower inflammation and improve general wellness.

Hydration and detoxification: stressing the need for sufficient hydration and foods that support the body's natural detoxification processes in order to achieve optimum health.

Foundations of healing nutrition

Healing nutrition refers to ideas and methods that use food to support health, energy, and overall wellbeing. These fundamental ideas center on providing the body with nourishment, facilitating the body's inherent healing abilities, and maximizing general health results. The following are the main tenets of healing nutrition:

Whole, nutrient-dense foods: to obtain vital vitamins, minerals, fiber, and antioxidants, prioritize unprocessed foods such as fruits, vegetables, whole grains, legumes, nuts, seeds, and lean proteins.

Plant-based emphasis: to lower the risk of chronic disease and promote heart health, prioritize a diet high in plant foods due to their anti-inflammatory and antioxidant qualities.

Macronutrient balancing: make sure your diet of lipids, proteins, and carbs is balanced and adapted to your specific needs for hormone synthesis, cognitive function, cell repair, and long-term energy.

Hydration and detoxification: to support healthy kidney function, digestion, and body temperature regulation, stay properly hydrated with water and hydrating meals. Consume healthy fats from foods like avocados, nuts, seeds, olive oil, and fatty seafood to help maintain hormone balance, heart health, mental clarity, and control overweight.

Mindful eating: to boost connection with hunger and satiety signals, minimize stress- related eating, improve digestion, and practice awareness and appreciation of food. Nutrient density and bioavailability: to optimize nutrient absorption, select foods that are high in vitamins, minerals, and antioxidants and prepare them according to recipe instructions.

Customized approach: tailor dietary recommendations to individual health concerns, preferences, and lifestyles for personalized and sustainable nutrition plans.

Adopting these principles helps individuals achieve optimal health, resilience, and vitality by supporting the body's natural healing processes and promoting long-term well-being.

The core principles of dr. O'Neill's nutritional teachings

D r. Barbara O'Neill emphasizes natural, plant-based diet and lifestyle practices to support optimal well-being in her nutritional teachings, which are based on holistic health principles. An in-depth examination of each tenet is provided below:

Plant-based diet: dr. O'neill promotes a diet high in whole grains, nuts, seeds, legumes, and colorful fruits and vegetables that are primarily plant-based. Essential vitamins, minerals, antioxidants, and phytochemicals found in these foods promote general health. Because plant-based diets are high in fiber and nutrient density, they are linked to a lower risk of chronic diseases like diabetes, heart disease, and some types of cancer.

Raw and whole foods: the idea that raw and minimally processed whole foods retain more of their natural enzymes, vitamins, and minerals is the foundation for the emphasis on these foods. It is believed that eating raw foods aids in digestion and nutrient absorption. Raw salads, fresh fruits, and sprouted grains are a few examples. These foods are thought to promote optimal health by supplying nutrients in their most natural, easily digestible form.

Alkaline balance: dr. O'Neill advocates for an alkaline-forming diet, placing special emphasis on foods that help the body maintain a slightly alkaline ph. Leafy greens, citrus fruits, and vegetables are examples of alkaline foods that are thought to support cellular health and lower inflammation. It is believed that this dietary strategy will help the body's inherent detoxification mechanisms and the immune system as a whole.

Hydration: Dr. O'Neill stresses the importance of staying properly hydrated in his lessons on preserving good health. She suggests drinking purified water all day long to help with detoxification, cellular hydration, and the healthy operation of body systems. Hydration aids in toxin removal, lubricating joints, supplying nutrients to cells, and controlling body temperature.

Detoxification: another important tenet of Dr. O'neill's nutritional philosophy is to support the body's natural detoxification processes. This is ingesting foods and liquids that support liver function and improve the detoxification process. Cruciferous vegetables (broccoli, cabbage), garlic, turmeric, and herbal teas with liver-supporting qualities are a few examples.

Dr. O'neill places a strong emphasis on selecting foods that are high in vitamins, minerals, and antioxidants in relation to their calorie content. This is known as nutrient density. Berries, whole grains, nuts, seeds, and dark leafy greens are examples of foods high in nutrients. These foods promote general health and vitality and help maximize nutritional intake.

Balanced diet: dr. O'Neill emphasizes the significance of a balanced diet while supporting a plant-based diet. To guarantee sufficient consumption of vital nutrients like protein, healthy fats (from sources like avocado and olive oil), carbohydrates (from whole grains and vegetables), vitamins, and minerals, a range of foods must be included. Maintaining a balance between macro and micronutrients promotes general health and guards against dietary deficiencies.

Holistic approach: Dr. O'Neill's dietary advice is a component of a holistic approach to health that takes into account how the body, mind, and spirit are all interconnected. She highlights the significance of proper diet in addition to stress reduction methods, consistent exercise, enough sleep, and mental health. The goal of this holistic approach is to promote overall wellness by addressing the underlying causes of health problems.

People can adopt a lifestyle that promotes maximum health, longevity, and vitality by adhering to these principles. The holistic nutritional teachings of Dr. Barbara O'Neill offers a framework for making educated food decisions and fostering general well-being using organic and sustainable methods.

BOOK 20:

Energizing Breakfast Recipes

Energizing breakfast recipes

Start your day with one of our nutrient-dense, energy-boosting meals that include protein, fiber, and antioxidants.

Avocado and smoked salmon toast

Ingredients:

2 slices whole grain bread, toasted 1 ripe avocado, mashed

100g smoked salmon 1 tbsp lemon juice

Salt and pepper to taste Fresh dill for garnish

Instructions:

In a bowl, beat the eggs and add the salt and pepper.

In a skillet over medium heat, warm the olive oil.

Add cherry tomatoes, onions, and bell peppers.

Sauté the veggies until they are soft. Add the eggs and scramble them until they are cooked through.

Greek yogurt and berry parfait

Ingredients:

200g greek yogurt

1 cup mixed berries (blueberries, strawberries, raspberries)

2 tbsp honey 1/4 cup granola

Instructions:

Arrange greek yogurt, granola, honey, and mixed berries in a glass.

Layers should be added until the glass is full. Serve right away.

Spinach and feta omelette

Ingredients:

3 large eggs

1 cup fresh spinach, chopped 1/4 cup feta cheese, crumbled Salt and pepper to taste

1 tbsp olive oil

Instructions:

In a bowl, beat the eggs and add the salt and pepper.

In a nonstick skillet, warm the olive oil over medium heat.

When the spinach begins to wilt, add it.

Add the eggs and heat until they are just set.

After covering one half of the omelet with feta cheese, fold the other half over.

Cook the eggs until they are set through.

Chia seed pudding with fresh fruit

Ingredients:

1/4 cup chia seeds 1 cup almond milk 1 tbsp maple syrup

Fresh fruit (e.g., kiwi, mango, berries)

Instructions:

In a bowl, mix chia seeds, almond milk, and maple syrup.

Stir well and refrigerate overnight.

In the morning, stir the pudding again and top with fresh fruit.

Banana and nut butter smoothie

Ingredients:

1 ripe banana

1 cup unsweetened almond milk

2 tbsp natural peanut butter or almond butter

1 tbsp honey

1/2 tsp cinnamon Ice cubes (optional)

Instructions:

Combine all ingredients in a blender. Blend until smooth.

Serve immediately.

Whole grain pancakes with fresh berries

Ingredients:

1 cup whole wheat flour 1 tbsp baking powder

1 tbsp honey

1 cup almond milk 1 large egg

1 cup fresh berries (blueberries, strawberries)

1 tbsp coconut oil

Instructions:

Combine the flour and baking powder in a bowl.

Combine the egg, almond milk, and honey in a separate bowl.

Stir the dry and wet ingredients together until smooth.

In a skillet over medium heat, preheat the coconut oil.

Transfer batter into skillet and cook until bubbles appear on top of the pancakes.

Cook till golden brown after flipping. Accompany with raw berries.

Savory quinoa breakfast bowl

Ingredients:

1 cup cooked quinoa 1/2 avocado, sliced

1/2 cup cherry tomatoes, halved 1 poached egg

1 tbsp olive oil

Salt and pepper to taste

Fresh herbs (e.g., cilantro, parsley)

Instructions:

Arrange cooked quinoa in a bowl. Topwith avocado slices, cherry tomatoes, and the poached egg.

Drizzle with olive oil and season with salt and pepper.

Garnish with fresh herbs.

Cottage cheese and tomato toast

Ingredients:

2 slices whole grain bread, toasted 1 cup cottage cheese

1 medium tomato, sliced Salt and pepper to taste

Fresh basil leaves

Instructions:

Spread cottage cheese evenly on the toasted bread.

Top with tomato slices. Season with salt and pepper. Garnish with fresh basil leaves.

Oatmeal with nuts and seeds

Ingredients:

1 cup rolled oats

2 cups water or milk

1/4 cup mixed nuts (almonds, walnuts)

1/4 cup mixed seeds (chia, flax, sunflower)

1 tbsp honey

1/2 tsp cinnamon

Instructions:

In a pot, bring water or milk to a boil. Add oats and reduce heat to simmer. Cook until oats are tender.

Stir in nuts, seeds, honey, and cinnamon. Serve warm.

Scrambled eggs with vegetables

Ingredients:

3 large eggs

1/4 cup bell peppers, diced 1/4 cup onions, diced

1/4 cup cherry tomatoes, halved Salt and pepper to taste

1 tbsp olive oil

Instructions:

In a bowl, beat the eggs and add the salt and pepper.

In a skillet over medium heat, warm the olive oil.

Add cherry tomatoes, onions, and bell peppers. Sauté the veggies until they are soft. Add the eggs and scramble them until they are cooked through.

Kale and mushroom tofu scramble

Ingredients:

1 block of firm tofu 350g

4 5 chestnut mushrooms â?? Sliced A generous handful of chopped kale

1 2 cloves of garlic

2 tbsp of nutritional yeast

A pinch of black salt for that eggy flavor or normal salt

1/2 tsp of turmeric

A crack of black pepper

Instructions:

When the mushrooms have shrunk in size, and the water has drained, add them to a skillet with a small amount of water and simmer for three to four minutes.

Stir in the smashed garlic after adding it.

Incorporate the chopped greens and blend everything thoroughly.

Crumble the tofu block with your hands.

Cook for three to four minutes after adding the nutritional yeast.

Lastly, include the turmeric and salt, blending well.

Serve with additional vegetables, bread, avocado, or whatever else you like!

Nutty banana smoothie

Ingredients:

1 banana, sliced and frozen 1/2 cup of milk of choice

2 tbsp peanut butter, be generous 2 tbsp greek yogurt, optional

Instructions:

Mix all ingredients until smooth.

Oatmeal with pumpkin seeds and pears

Ingredients:

80g oats

2 tbsp quinoa

2 tbsp chia seeds 360ml plant-based milk

2 tsp diy pumpkin pie spice blend Cinnamon pears:

6 pears

1 tsp cinnamon

2 tbsp coconut sugar To serve:

2 tbsp vegan yoghurt 2 tbsp almond butter 1 handful raspberries

Instructions:

Preheat the oven to 160°fan/180°c in order to prepare the cinnamon pears. Pears should be sliced, seeded, and chopped into 1 cm pieces. Mix in 2 tablespoons coconut sugar and 1 tsp cinnamon. Bake for 20 minutes in an ovenproof dish or until soft and gooey.

Make the pumpkin pie spice overnight oats by combining the oats, quinoa, chia seeds, plant-based milk, and spices. Store the mixture in a covered container and let it sit overnight to become thick and creamy.

Garnish the oats with almond butter, raspberries, vegan yogurt, and cinnamon-pears.

Overnight oats with almond butter and raspberry

Ingredients:

½ cup (63 g) raspberries, fresh or frozen

½ tablespoon lemon juice

½ cup (45 g) old-fashioned rolled oats

½ cup (118 ml) dairy-free milk

1 tablespoon almond butter

1 tablespoon ground flax seed

½ tablespoon maple syrup

¼ teaspoon vanilla extract Toppings

Cocoa nibs or vegan chocolate chips Sliced almonds

Dairy-free yogurt Fresh raspberries Oil-free granola Coconut flakes

Instructions:

In order to maintain the color of the raspberries, mash them at the bottom of the jar and add ½ tablespoon of lemon juice. Before mashing frozen raspberries, let them thaw slightly and then squeeze in ½ spoonful of lemon juice.

Next, combine the raspberries with the oats, milk, almond butter, crushed flaxseed, syrup, and vanilla extract.

Mix everything together.

To make it thicker, cover and refrigerate for two to three hours or overnight.

Keep for two to three days.

Quinoa breakfast bowl with almonds and berries

Ingredients:

1/4 cup uncooked pre-washed quinoa, or rinse well under water

1/2 cup unsweetened almond milk 1/2 teaspoon cinnamon

1/2 teaspoon vanilla extract 2 tsp honey

1 medium banana, sliced 6 strawberries, sliced 1/2 cup blueberries

2 tsp hemp seeds, pepitas or nuts 1/4 cup warmed almond milk

Instructions:

Pour the almond milk, cinnamon, and vanilla into a small saucepan, bring to a boil, then lower the heat to a simmer. Add the quinoa, cover, and cook on low for 20 to 25 minutes or until the liquid is gone.

Using a fork, fluff.

Split the heated quinoa between two bowls, then top with hemp seeds and sliced fruit. Drizzle with honey and, if preferred, top with warm milk.

Spiced apple porridge

Ingredients:

250g peeled and cubed bramley apple (about 3 medium apples)

1 tbsp honey

1 tsp ground cinnamon

½ tsp ground ginger

1 good pinch of freshly grated nutmeg 1 pinch salt

70g porridge oats

300ml oat drink (or whole milk) 50ml water

40g sultanas

1 handful granola Natural yogurt

Instructions:

In a skillet over low heat, combine 250g of peeled and diced bramley apples (approximately 3 medium apples), 1 tbsp honey, 1 tsp ground cinnamon, ½ tsp powdered ginger, and a generous sprinkling of salt and freshly grated nutmeg. When the apple starts to soften, cook it covered for four to five minutes (if it seems dry, add a splash of water).

Remove half of the apple mixture and use the back of a fork to mash the remaining portion softly in the pan. To the apples, add 70g porridge oats, 300ml oat drink (or whole milk), 50ml water, and 40g sultanas. Cook over low heat until the oats are tender and the consistency you want, around 7 to 8 minutes.

Spoon into two dishes; sprinkle with a handful of granola and the leftover cooked apples. Also excellent is a small amount of natural yogurt.

Spinach and avocado smoothie

Ingredients:

1 cup nonfat plain yogurt 1 cup fresh spinach

1 frozen banana

¼ avocado

2 tablespoons water

1 teaspoon honey

Instructions:

In a blender, combine yogurt, spinach, banana, avocado, water, and honey. Blend until smooth.

Sweet potato and black bean breakfast burritos.

Ingredients:

1 yellow onion, diced

3 medium to large sweet potatoes, peeled and diced

1 cup black beans (rinse and drain if using canned)

1 cup salsa of choice

2 cup fresh spinach Wraps of choice

Optional: parchment paper for wrapping

Instructions:

Wash, cut, and dice every vegetable. In a big skillet or saucepan, combine the sweet potatoes and diced onion with 1/3 cup of water. For five to seven minutes, cook with a lid on over medium-high heat.

Take off the pan's top, turn down the heat to medium, and add the salsa and black beans. If needed, add a little water as well. After stirring and covering, boil the sweet potatoes for ten to fifteen minutes or until they are soft. Take off the heat and place aside. Once the combination of sweet potatoes and beans has cooled down enough to handle, assemble your burritos using your preferred wrapper.

To each wrapper, add a tiny handful of fresh spinach, if preferred. Place a piece of parchment paper over each burrito and keep it in the refrigerator for up to six days or the freezer for up to thirty.

Just pop the burritos in the microwave for two to three minutes to reheat and defrost. Accompany with more guacamole, hummus, or salsa.

Zucchini bread oatmeal

Ingredients:

For the oatmeal:

1 (14-ounce/400 ml) can light coconut milk

2/3 cup (66 g) gluten-free rolled oats*

1 cup (125 g) packed finely grated zucchini (1 medium)

2 tablespoons (20 g) chia seeds

1/2 to 1 teaspoon cinnamon, to taste 1/4 teaspoon freshly grated nutmeg or a dash of ground nutmeg

1 1/2 tablespoons (22.5 ml) pure maple syrup or 1 large ripe banana, mashed

Small pinch of fine sea salt

1 teaspoon pure vanilla extract Topping suggestions:

Chopped pecans

Raisins or chopped pitted dates Pat of coconut oil or vegan butter Pure maple syrup or coconut sugar Cinnamon

Shaved dark chocolate

Instructions:

In a medium saucepan, add all the oatmeal ingredients (except the vanilla) and whisk to mix. Place mixture over medium-high heat and bring to a simmer. Turn down the heat to medium. Simmer, uncovered, stirring constantly, for 7 to 9 minutes or until thickened.

After taking off the heat, whisk in the vanilla. If desired, taste and adjust the sugar and spices.

After dividing the oats into bowls, add the toppings of your choice. Store leftovers in the refrigerator for three to five days in an airtight container. Place the leftovers in a small saucepan with a little coconut milk to reheat. Stir and cook on medium until well cooked. As an alternative, you may also eat leftovers cold!

BOOK 21:

Revitalizing Lunches Recipes

Revitalizing lunches recipes

Avocado quinoa salad with lemon dressing

Ingredients:

Salad

2 cups cooked quinoa

1 pound Persian or English cucumbers

2 large avocados peeled and chopped 6 green onions finely chopped

1 handful fresh parsley leaves finely chopped

½ cup chopped walnuts Dressing

⅓ cup fresh lemon juice or the juice of two lemons

3 tablespoons extra virgin olive oil 2 cloves garlic

2 large medjool dates Salt to taste

Instructions:

Place the cooked quinoa and cucumbers in a large salad dish. Add the green onions and avocados and mix. Finally, stir in the walnuts and parsley; put aside.

To make the dressing, put all the ingredients in a blender and pulse until everything is mashed and the consistency is creamy, about a few seconds. Savor and pass the dressing alongside.

Baked sweet potato and hummus wrap

Ingredients:

1 medium sweet potato, peeled and cut into 1" cubes

1 tablespoon olive oil

½ teaspoon fine sea salt

¼ teaspoon black pepper

1 can chickpeas, drained and rinsed 1 tablespoon tahini

1 garlic clove, chopped

2 tablespoons lemon juice 1 teaspoon fine sea salt

½ teaspoon black pepper

¼ cup olive oil

4 tumaro's 8" garden veggie carb wise wraps

1 package (5oz) baby spinach

1 cucumber, peeled and thinly sliced

½ cup jarred roasted red bell peppers, drained and thinly sliced

½ cup sprouts, such as broccoli or radish sprouts

½ cup almonds, toasted and chopped

Instructions:

Turn the oven on to 400°f.

On a baking pan, spread the sweet potatoes out. Season with salt, pepper, and olive oil. Bake for approximately 20 minutes or until soft and gently browned. Place aside and allow to cool.

Roasted potatoes, chickpeas, tahini, garlic, lemon juice, salt, and pepper should all be combined in a food processor. To blend, pulse. Olive oil should be added steadily while the machine is operating. Process till well combined. If necessary, taste and add more salt and pepper.

Place a quarter cup of hummus in the middle of every wrapper. Add sprouts, almonds, roasted pepper, cucumber, spinach, and sprouts on top. If desired, tuck the edges of the wrap in, fold the bottom of the wrap over the filling, and securely roll up. Divide in two.

Beetroot and spinach salad with walnuts

Ingredients:

2 large beets, trimmed 8 ounces baby spinach

1/3 cup crumbled goat cheese 1/2 cup toasted walnuts

2 tablespoons extra-virgin olive oil 1 tablespoon red wine vinegar Scant 1/2 teaspoon salt

1/4 teaspoon pepper

Instructions:

Aim for 425°f (220°c) in the oven. On a baking

sheet, arrange the beets. Depending on the size of the beets, roast for approximately an hour or until fork tender. Peel and coarsely slice beets after they're cold enough to handle. In a large bowl, combine spinach, beets, goat cheese, and walnuts.

Mix the vinegar and olive oil in a small bowl. Add the pepper and salt and whisk. Drizzle salad with dressing and toss to mix.

Black bean taco salad with cilantro-lime dressing

Ingredients:

Tortilla bowls 6 large tortillas

4 tablespoons vegetable oil Creamy cilantro lime dressing 2 cups cilantro stems included

½ cup sour cream

¼ cup olive oil (or mayonnaise)

½ teaspoon minced garlic

½ teaspoon ground coriander

½ teaspoon salt more if needed

½ jalapeno diced (optional) 2 limes, juiced

Taco salad ingredients 1 pound ground beef

1 (1-ounce package) taco seasoning 1 cup corn (canned, frozen or fresh)

6 cups shredded lettuce 2-3 romaine heads

1 cup diced tomatoes

½ cup sliced black olives, optional 1 cup canned black beans rinsed

½ cup sour cream

1 avocado sliced or 1 cup guacamole

1 cup shredded Mexican blend cheese 1 cup salsa

¼ cup white or red onion diced 1 lime sliced, optional

1 cup corn chips doritos, corn chips, tortilla chips

6 taco bowls Instructions Taco bowls

Set oven temperature to 350°.

Instructions:

Heat up a big skillet and pour in one spoonful of oil. Cook a tortilla until it begins to bubble, then turn it over and allow it to bubble again.

Take it out and put it in a bowl, carefully pressing down so as not to tear the tortilla while maintaining the edges raised or turn the bowl over and place it on top of the bowl, pressing down on the sides to ensure the bowl is covered.

After setting the bowls on a baking sheet, bake them for fifteen minutes. Before removing, tap the tortillas to ensure they are nice and crisp. Check the doneness after a minute or two of baking if the bottoms are not crispy enough.

Creamy cilantro lime dressing

In a food processor, combine the sour cream, garlic, coriander, olive oil, and cilantro; process until smooth.

Stir together the minced jalapeño and the lime juice.

Taco salad

Place the meat and taco seasoning in a pan. Once the meat is cooked through, add the corn and let it softly brown.

Add the lettuce first, followed by the tomatoes, if you're using taco bowls. Add the onion, salsa, sour cream, avocado, cheese, beans, and olive. If you'd like, you may squeeze in some fresh lime juice.

After adding the dressing, serve.

In case taco bowls are not available, arrange the salad in a bowl and then top each bowl with chips and dressing.

Broccoli and almond soup

Ingredients:

50 g ground almonds 650 g broccoli

1 litre water

1 stock cube To season:

Salt & pepper (optional) Fresh herbs (optional)

Instructions:

Warm up a substantial frying pan. Avoid adding any oil and let it get "dry" before rapidly frying the powdered almonds until they are golden brown.

Stir them frequently since they may burn quickly.

To prevent them from cooking any longer, turn

them out onto a platter after they have toasted.

Cut the broccoli into little pieces and place it in a big pot with some water and a crumbled stock cube.

Bring the mixture quickly to a boil, then lower the heat and simmer the broccoli for 8 to 10 minutes, or until it becomes soft.

To make the soup smooth and creamy, add the toasted ground almonds to the pan, swirl, and mix.

After tasting the soup, determine if it needs extra spice.

Add some salt if you think it tastes a little bland.

Add a pinch of freshly ground black pepper for extra heat.

Divide the soup into four dishes or meal prep containers, and garnish with fresh herbs, if preferred.

Enjoy with some crusty bread!

Chickpea and avocado sandwich on sprouted bread

Ingredients:

1 can no salt added chickpeas drained and rinsed

1 large ripe avocado1

½ tbsp lemon juice

½ tsp hot chili pepper finely minced Salt and pepper

4 slices whole grain sprouted bread 1 large heirloom tomato sliced

½ cup sweet microgreens

½ cup shredded carrot

½ cup cooked and shredded beet

Instructions:

Mash the avocado fairly smooth in a bowl, then stir in the chickpeas, lemon juice, and spicy chile pepper. Add pepper and salt for seasoning.

To create the sandwich, place one slice of bread with the tomato slices on it, then top with the carrots, beets, chickpea salad, and microgreens. Cut into the rogue and savor!

Cold lentil salad with sun-dried tomatoes

Ingredients:

2 cups cooked lentils (or a little more if you use a slightly larger package of pre-cooked lentils)

1-8.5-ounce jar sun-dried tomatoes in olive oil, julienne sliced

3 tablespoons lemon juice (about one lemon)

1 clove garlic, minced

1 cup fresh parsley, chopped

Salt and pepper, to taste (optional)

Instructions:

The lentils should be put in a big salad dish.

To the bowl, add three tablespoons of the olive oil from the sun-dried tomato container. After removing any leftover oil, include the sun-dried tomatoes.

Add the parsley, garlic, and lemon juice after that.

Make sure to give the lentils a good toss to coat them well in the olive oil.

If desired, add salt and pepper after tasting.

Serve right away or put in the fridge to enjoy later.

Cucumber noodle salad with peanut dressing

Ingredients:

1 whole english cucumber Garnish toasted sesame seeds Thai peanut sauce

¼ cup unsalted peanut butter, almond butter, or sun butter for nut-free

1-1.5 tsp red curry paste

¼ cup full-fat canned coconut milk

1.5 tbsp tamarind paste, or apple cider vinegar

⅛ tsp coarse sea salt 1 tbsp coconut water

Instructions:

Using a julienne peeler, thinly slice the cucumber till nearly to the core, which contains the seeds.

To drain excess moisture, spread the cucumber noodles out on a broad, flat platter covered with paper towels. While making the sauce, keep the noodles refrigerated.

Mix the ingredients (peanut butter and coconut water) in a measuring cup. Mix well and stir.

Spoon the sauce over the noodles after transferring them to a serving platter. Throw accurately. Serve right away cold.

Grilled chicken and quinoa salad

Ingredients:

1 cup cooked quinoa

200g grilled chicken breast, sliced 1 cup mixed greens

1/2 cup cherry tomatoes, halved 1/4 cup cucumber, diced

1/4 cup red onion, thinly sliced 2 tbsp olive oil

1 tbsp balsamic vinegar Salt and pepper to taste

Instructions:

In a large bowl, combine quinoa, mixed greens, cherry tomatoes, cucumber, and red onion.

Top with grilled chicken slices. Drizzle with olive oil and balsamic vinegar.

Season with salt and pepper and toss to combine.

Turkey and avocado wrap

Ingredients:

1 whole wheat tortilla 100g sliced turkey breast

1/2 avocado, sliced

1/4 cup shredded lettuce 1/4 cup sliced cucumber 1 tbsp hummus

Salt and pepper to taste

Instructions:

Spread hummus evenly on the tortilla. Layer turkey slices, avocado, lettuce, and cucumber.

Season with salt and pepper.

Roll up the tortilla tightly and slice it in half.

Salmon and asparagus stir-fry

Ingredients:

200g salmon fillet, cut into cubes

1 bunch asparagus, trimmed and cut into pieces

1 red bell pepper, sliced

1 clove garlic, minced

2 tbsp soy sauce 1 tbsp olive oil

1 tsp sesame oil

1 tsp fresh ginger, grated

Instructions:

Heat olive oil in a large skillet over medium heat.

Add garlic and ginger, and sauté for 1 minute.

Add salmon cubes and cook until lightly browned.

Add asparagus and red bell pepper, and stir-fry until vegetables are tender. Pour in soy sauce and sesame oil and stir to combine. Serve hot.

Mediterranean chickpea salad

Ingredients:

1 can chickpeas, drained and rinsed 1 cup cherry tomatoes, halved

1/2 cup cucumber, diced 1/4 cup red onion, diced

1/4 cup feta cheese, crumbled 2 tbsp olive oil

1 tbsp lemon juice

Salt and pepper to taste Fresh parsley, chopped

Instructions:

In a large bowl, combine chickpeas, cherry tomatoes, cucumber, red onion, and feta cheese. Drizzle with olive oil and lemon juice. Season with salt and pepper and toss to combine. Garnish with fresh parsley.

Spicy shrimp tacos

Ingredients:

200g shrimp, peeled and deveined 1 tsp chili powder

1/2 tsp cumin 1/2 tsp paprika

Salt and pepper to taste 1 tbsp olive oil

4 small corn tortillas

1/2 cup shredded cabbage 1/4 cup diced mango

1/4 cup diced red onion Fresh cilantro for garnish Lime wedges for serving

Instructions:

Combine the prawns, paprika, cumin, chili powder, and salt & pepper in a bowl.

In a skillet over medium heat, warm the olive oil.

Shrimp should be cooked thoroughly and pink.

In a dry skillet, reheat the tortillas. Stuff tortillas with red onion, mango, cabbage and prawns.

Serve with lime wedges and garnish with fresh cilantro.

Chicken and vegetable stir-fry

Ingredients:

200g chicken breast, thinly sliced 1 cup

broccoli florets

1 red bell pepper, sliced

1 carrot, julienned

2 tbsp soy sauce 1 tbsp olive oil 1 tsp sesame oil

1 clove garlic, minced

1 tsp fresh ginger, grated

Instructions:

Heat olive oil in a large skillet over medium heat.

Add garlic and ginger, and sauté for 1 minute.

Add chicken slices and cook until no longer pink.

Add broccoli, bell pepper, and carrot, and stir-fry until vegetables are tender.

Pour in soy sauce and sesame oil and stir to combine.

Serve hot.

Tuna and white bean salad

Ingredients:

1 can tuna, drained

1 can white beans, drained and rinsed 1/2
cup cherry tomatoes, halved

1/4 cup red onion, diced 2 tbsp olive oil

1 tbsp lemon juice

Salt and pepper to taste Fresh basil for
garnish

Instructions:

In a large bowl, combine tuna, white beans,
cherry tomatoes, and red onion.

Drizzle with olive oil and lemon juice. Season
with salt and pepper and toss to combine.

Garnish with fresh basil.

Beef and broccoli stir-fry

Ingredients:

200g beef sirloin, thinly sliced 1 cup broccoli
florets

1/2 red bell pepper, sliced

2 tbsp soy sauce 1 tbsp olive oil 1 tsp
sesame oil

1 clove garlic, minced

1 tsp fresh ginger, grated

Instructions:

In a big skillet over medium heat, warm up
the olive oil.

Add the ginger and garlic and cook for one
minute.

Cook the meat pieces until they get browned.
When the veggies are soft, add the bell pepper and
broccoli and stir-fry them. Add the sesame oil and
soy sauce, then whisk everything together.
Warm up the food.

Chicken and avocado salad

Ingredients:

200g grilled chicken breast, sliced 1 avocado,
sliced

1 cup mixed greens

1/2 cup cherry tomatoes, halved 1/4 cup red
onion, thinly sliced 2 tbsp olive oil

1 tbsp balsamic vinegar Salt and pepper to taste

Instructions:

In a large bowl, combine mixed greens, cherry

tomatoes, and red onion.

Top with grilled chicken slices and avocado.

Drizzle with olive oil and balsamic vinegar.

Season with salt and pepper and toss to combine.

Lentil and vegetable soup

Ingredients:

1 cup lentils, rinsed 1 carrot, diced

1 celery stalk, diced

1 onion, diced

2 cloves garlic, minced 1 can diced tomatoes

4 cups vegetable broth 1 tbsp olive oil

1 tsp cumin

1 tsp paprika

Salt and pepper to taste Fresh parsley for garnish

Instructions:

Heat olive oil in a large pot over medium heat.

Add onion, carrot, celery, and garlic, and

sauté until vegetables are tender. Add lentils, diced tomatoes, vegetable broth, cumin, and paprika.

Bring to a boil, then reduce heat and simmer for 20-25 minutes, until lentils are tender.

Season with salt and pepper.

Garnish with fresh parsley before serving.

BOOK 22:

Nourishing Dinners Recipes

Nourishing dinners recipes

Baked lemon herb chicken

Ingredients:

4 boneless, skinless chicken breasts

2 lemons, sliced

3 cloves garlic, minced

2 tbsp olive oil

1 tbsp dried oregano 1 tbsp dried thyme

Salt and pepper to taste Fresh parsley for garnish

Instructions:

Set oven temperature to 200°c, or 400°f.

Chicken breasts should be put on a baking dish.

Combine the olive oil, garlic, thyme, oregano, and salt & pepper in a small bowl.

Coat the chicken breasts with the mixture.

Add slices of lemon on top.

Bake the chicken for 25 to 30 minutes or until it is thoroughly done.

Before serving, garnish with fresh parsley.

Grilled salmon with avocado salsa

Ingredients:

4 salmon fillets 2 tbsp olive oil

Salt and pepper to taste 1 avocado, diced

1 tomato, diced

1/4 cup red onion, diced 1 lime, juiced

Fresh cilantro for garnish

Instructions:

Set the grill's temperature to medium- high.

Salmon fillets should be seasoned with salt and pepper and brushed with olive oil.

Seared salmon should be grilled for 4– 5 minutes on each side.

Combine avocado, tomato, red onion, and lime juice in a bowl.

Present the grilled salmon with avocado salsa on top.

Add fresh cilantro as a garnish.

Stuffed bell peppers

Ingredients:

4 bell peppers, tops cut off and seeds removed

200g ground turkey 1 cup cooked quinoa 1 cup diced tomatoes 1/2 cup corn kernels

1/2 cup black beans, drained and rinsed

1/2 cup shredded cheese 1 tsp cumin

1 tsp paprika

Salt and pepper to taste

Instructions:

Turn the oven on to 180°c, or 350°f. Cook the ground turkey in a pan until browned.

Add the chopped tomatoes, black beans, corn, cumin, paprika, cooked quinoa, and salt and pepper.

Place the mixture inside the bell peppers.

Top the peppers in a baking dish with cheddar that has been shredded.

Bake peppers for 25 to 30 minutes or until soft.

Shrimp and vegetable skewers

Ingredients:

200g shrimp, peeled and deveined 1 zucchini, sliced

1 red bell pepper, cut into chunks

1 yellow bell pepper, cut into chunks

1 red onion, cut into chunks

2 tbsp olive oil

1 tsp garlic powder 1 tsp paprika

Salt and pepper to taste

Instructions:

Preheat the grill to medium-high heat. In a bowl, toss shrimp and vegetables with olive oil, garlic powder, paprika, salt, and pepper.

Thread shrimp and vegetables onto skewers.

Grill for 3-4 minutes per side until shrimp are pink and vegetables are tender.

Spaghetti squash with meat sauce

Ingredients:

1 large spaghetti squash 200g ground beef

1 can diced tomatoes

1 small onion, diced

2 cloves garlic, minced 1 tbsp olive oil

1 tsp dried basil

1 tsp dried oregano Salt and pepper to taste

Fresh basil for garnish

Instructions:

Set oven temperature to 200°c, or 400°f.

Remove the seeds after cutting the spaghetti squash in half lengthwise.

Apply a thin layer of olive oil and sprinkle with salt and pepper.

After placing the halves of the squash cut-side down on a baking pan, bake for 40 to 45 minutes.

Cook ground beef till browned in a pan.

Add the garlic and onion and cook until soft.

Add salt, pepper, dried oregano, dried basil, and diced tomatoes.

Allow to simmer for fifteen minutes. Scrape out the spaghetti squash strands with a fork.

Spoon the spaghetti squash with the beef sauce.

Throw some fresh basil on top.

Chicken and broccoli stir-fry

Ingredients:

200g chicken breast, thinly sliced 2 cups broccoli florets

1 red bell pepper, sliced

2 cloves garlic, minced 2 tbsp soy sauce

1 tbsp olive oil 1 tsp sesame oil

1 tsp fresh ginger, grated

Instructions:

Heat olive oil in a large skillet over medium heat.

Add garlic and ginger, and sauté for 1 minute.

Add chicken slices and cook until no longer pink.

Add broccoli and bell pepper, and stir- fry until vegetables are tender.

Pour in soy sauce and sesame oil and stir to combine.

Serve hot.

Baked cod with mediterranean vegetables

Ingredients:

4 cod fillets

1 zucchini, sliced

1 yellow squash, sliced 1 red bell pepper, sliced

1 red onion, sliced

2 tbsp olive oil

1 tsp dried oregano 1 tsp dried thyme

Salt and pepper to taste Lemon wedges for serving

Instructions:

Preheat the oven to 200°c (400°f). Place cod fillets in a baking dish and arrange vegetables around them.

Drizzle with olive oil and season with oregano, thyme, salt, and pepper.

Bake for 20-25 minutes, until the fish is opaque and vegetables are tender.

Serve with lemon wedges.

Beef and vegetable stir- fry

Ingredients:

200g beef sirloin, thinly sliced 1 cup snap peas

1 red bell pepper, sliced

1 carrot, julienned

2 tbsp soy sauce 1 tbsp olive oil 1 tsp sesame oil

1 clove garlic, minced

1 tsp fresh ginger, grated

Instructions:

Heat olive oil in a large skillet over medium heat.

Add garlic and ginger, and sauté for 1 minute.

Add beef slices and cook until browned.

Add snap peas, bell pepper, and carrot, and stir-fry until vegetables are tender.

Pour in soy sauce and sesame oil and stir to combine.

Serve hot.

Herb-crusted pork tenderloin

Ingredients:

1 pork tenderloin

2 tbsp olive oil

2 cloves garlic, minced

1 tbsp fresh rosemary, chopped 1 tbsp fresh thyme, chopped Salt and pepper to taste

Instructions:

Preheat the oven to 200°c (400°f). Rub the pork tenderloin with olive oil, garlic, rosemary, thyme, salt, and pepper.

Place in a baking dish and roast for 25-

30 minutes, until the internal temperature reaches 63°c (145°f).

Let rest for 5 minutes before slicing.

Chicken and vegetable skewers

Ingredients:

200g chicken breast, cut into chunks 1 zucchini, sliced

1 red bell pepper, cut into chunks

1 yellow bell pepper, cut into chunks

1 red onion, cut into chunks

2 tbsp olive oil

1 tsp garlic powder 1 tsp paprika

Salt and pepper to taste

Instructions:

Preheat the grill to medium-high heat. In a bowl, toss chicken and vegetables with olive oil, garlic powder, paprika, salt, and pepper.

Thread chicken and vegetables onto skewers.

Grill for 8-10 minutes, turning occasionally, until chicken is cooked through.

Almond-crusted baked tofu

Ingredients:

Tofu

1 16-oz block tofu, 453 g

1 tbsp sesame oil, 15 ml

1 tbsp olive oil, 15 ml, or just 2 tbsp olive oil if you don't have sesame

2 tbsp reduced sodium soy sauce, 30 ml

1 clove garlic, minced Breading

¼ cup flour, 31 g, or all-purpose gluten-free flour

1 egg, or 1 tbsp ground flax seed + 3 tbsp water for vegan, whisked

1 cup whole almonds, 170 g 1 tbsp nutritional yeast

½ tsp salt

½ tsp paprika

¼ tsp ground black pepper Dipping sauce

1 avocado

½ cup plain Greek yogurt, 142 g, or dairy-free alternative

½ cup fresh chopped parsley, a handful

2 cloves garlic, minced Juice of 1 lime

Pinch each of salt and pepper

Instructions:

After draining, cut the tofu into 1" x 1" x ½" chunks. To absorb extra moisture, place a couple layers of paper towels on top and gently press with more. Tofu blocks should be placed in a deep dish (such as a storage container).

Mix together the soy sauce, sesame oil, olive oil, and chopped garlic. Cover and allow the tofu to sit in the marinade for at least half an hour, preferably longer. Turn the container occasionally to allow all of the tofu to become coated in the delicious marinade.

Grind almonds roughly by hand or in a food processor. Add black pepper, paprika, nutritional yeast, and salt and mix.

Set up your breading station by dividing the ingredients into three bowls: flour, egg, and almond mixture. Place a baking sheet coated with parchment paper in the last bowl. Shake off any leftover marinade from the tofu blocks, then place one or two at a time on a baking sheet and lightly cover each in flour, egg, and almond mixture.

Bake tofu nuggets for 8 to 10 minutes, turning halfway through, or until toasted and golden brown at 400 degrees fahrenheit (204 degrees celsius).

Place all the ingredients for the dipping sauce in a food processor and mix until smooth and creamy while the nuggets are cooking. Garnish the nuggets with heated dipping sauce.

Barley and vegetable stew

Ingredients:

1 yellow onion

2 cloves garlic 2 tbsp olive oil

1/2 lb. Carrots (about 4)

1 28oz. Can diced tomatoes 1 cup pearled barley

1/2 tsp dried basil 1/2 tsp dried oregano

Freshly cracked black pepper 6 cups vegetable broth

1 russet potato (about 3/4 lb.) 1 cup frozen green beans

1/2 cup frozen corn 1/2 cup frozen peas 1 tbsp lemon juice

1 handful fresh parsley (optional garnish)

Instructions:

Chop the garlic and dice the onion. Put the onion, garlic, and olive oil in a big soup pot and cook over medium heat until the onion becomes soft and transparent, about 5 minutes.

Peel and chop the carrots in the meanwhile. When the onions are

tender, add the carrots to the soup pot together with the vegetable broth, barley, basil, oregano, canned diced tomatoes with their juices, and some freshly cracked pepper.

After giving the pot a good stir and covering it, increase the heat to medium-high and boil the soup. After the soup reaches a boil, reduce the heat to medium-low and simmer it for

30 minutes while covering it and stirring now and again.

Peel and cut the potato into 1/2-inch pieces

while the soup is simmering. Add the diced potatoes and boil for a further 10 minutes, or until the potatoes are just tender, after the soup has simmered and the barley is almost soft.

Add the frozen green beans, corn, and peas after the potatoes are soft. After combining and heating thoroughly, stir (the soup should simmer for around 5 minutes).

Lastly, pour the lemon juice into the soup and mix everything together. After tasting the soup, taste and add more salt or pepper as needed. If preferred, sprinkle freshly chopped parsley over the top before serving hot.

Broccoli almond stir-fry

Ingredients:

5 cups broccoli florets 1 tablespoon canola oil

½ teaspoon minced garlic

2 tablespoons low-sodium soy sauce 1 tablespoon sugar

¼ teaspoon ground ginger

1 teaspoon fresh lemon juice

¼ cup slivered almonds toasted

Instructions:

Stir-fry broccoli in oil for 2 minutes, or until crisp-tender, in a nonstick pan or wok.

Fried garlic for one minute after adding it. Ginger, sugar, and soy sauce should be added. Cook for one to two minutes or until the sugar is dissolved. After adding almonds and lemon juice, serve.

Butternut squash soup with sage

Ingredients:

1 butternut squash, about 2 cups cubed

1 carrot, peeled

1 small onion, chopped 1 celery rib, chopped

6 cups of fat-free chicken or vegetable broth

2 garlic cloves, halved 4 sage leaves

1/2 cup 1% milk

Salt and freshly ground pepper

Instructions:

Squash should be peeled and the seeds removed.

Cut into cubes of a reasonable size. (Chopping

off the top and bottom of the butternut squash makes peeling it the simplest. Cut the squash lengthwise after that.)

Bring the broth, squash, carrots, celery, onion, garlic, and sage to a boil in a big, heavy saucepan. Squash should be cooked for about 40 minutes on low heat, covered, and simmering.

After discarding the sage, purée the soup using an immersion blender.

After adding the milk, taste and adjust the salt and pepper, and serve. Wonderful with freshly grated parmesan cheese on top.

Cauliflower steaks with herb sauce

Ingredients:

Lemon-herb sauce

1 cup parsley leaves

½ cup cilantro leaves

½ cup mint leaves

½ cup roughly chopped green onion 1 garlic

clove, smashed

Juice of 1 lemon

⅓ cup olive oil Cauliflower steaks

1 large head of cauliflower

4 tablespoons extra-virgin olive oil, divided

4 teaspoons smoked paprika

Salt and freshly ground black pepper to taste

Instructions:

To make the herb sauce, puree the parsley, cilantro, mint, green onion, garlic, lemon juice, and olive oil in a food processor or blender until very smooth. Put aside.

Prepare the steaks of cauliflower: slice the cauliflower into 1-inch-thick pieces using a sharp knife. (Around eight slices should come out.) Take roughly a teaspoon of olive oil and rub it on both sides of each cauliflower slice. Season each piece on both sides with salt, pepper, and a ½ teaspoon of smoky paprika.

In a large cast-iron pan, heat the remaining 1 tablespoon of olive oil over medium-high heat. Sear the cauliflower steaks in batches for three to four minutes on each side, or until they are golden brown. A fork should be able to readily penetrate the cauliflower, but it shouldn't be so soft that it crumbles.

To serve, arrange two cauliflower steaks on each dish and sprinkle a good amount of the herb-lemon sauce over them. Serve right away.

Chickpea and spinach curry

Ingredient:

1 tablespoon coconut oil

1 large onion or 2 regular (optional for a thicker sauce) finely diced

3 garlic cloves, minced

400 grams cherry tomatoes, halved approx 2 punnets

teaspoon garam masala

1-1 ½ teaspoon curry powder; add more for more heat

½ teaspoon turmeric

½ teaspoon ground cinnamon

¼ teaspoon ground cardamom

½ teaspoon ground cumin

½ teaspoon sea salt plus more to taste

½ teaspoon grated ginger 1 tablespoon tomato paste

480 grams cooked chickpeas cooked or 2 cans (drained)

200 ml coconut milk, half a 400ml (14 oz) can

¾ cup vegetable stock or water 3 cups baby spinach

1 teaspoon chili flakes or diced green chilies to serve (optional)

Instructions:

In a heavy-bottomed saucepan over medium heat, melt the coconut oil, add the onion, and simmer for three to five minutes or until tender. Add the tomatoes and garlic.

Add the ginger, tomato paste, turmeric, cinnamon, cardamom, cumin, garam masala, curry powder, and sea salt. Simmer for two minutes. Stir to coat after adding the chickpeas. After adding the coconut milk and vegetable stock, heat the blend until it boils.

Lower the temperature to low and let the pot uncovered while cooking for about 25 to 30 minutes, or until the sauce thickens and becomes creamy. Add the baby spinach and toss to slightly wilt.

Take the curry off the stove and serve it over cooked rice or quinoa and a sprinkle of chilli flakes or chiles.

Grilled asparagus and quinoa salad

Ingredients:

1 cup cooked quinoa

½ cup red bell pepper diced

½ cup red onions diced

2 tbsp chives

1 cup roasted asparagus diagonally cut Salt and pepper to taste

1/3 cup homemade vinaigrette

Instructions:

Combine all the ingredients, excluding the prepared vinaigrette, in a large bowl.

Toss to mix all the ingredients.

Next, drizzle the salad with the vinaigrette and give it a good toss.

If you believe it's required, adjust the seasoning by tasting it.

Herbed mushroom and quinoa risotto

Ingredients:

5 cups of water, bring to a boil 2 tbsp extra virgin olive oil

1 tsp crushed red pepper

2 shallots, finely chopped

3 cloves garlic, chopped

15 ounces baby bella mushrooms, sliced

1 cup organic white quinoa, rinsed 1/2 cup white wine

1/2 cup manchego cheese, grated 8-10 chives,

chopped

1 tbsp white truffle oil

Salt to taste

1/4 tsp black pepper

Instructions:

In a saucepan, bring the water to a boil. This will be used to finish cooking the quinoa and risotto with mushrooms.

Slice the mushrooms and finely chop the shallots and garlic.

Add extra virgin olive oil to a saucepan that has been heated over medium heat. Add the crushed red pepper right away, and allow it to sear for a few seconds.

Saute the shallots and garlic together for around two minutes.

Sliced mushrooms should be added. Give the mushrooms around ten minutes to cook. During this period, they will leak some water.

This is what you should eat when the mushrooms have cooked down. Add salt to taste to season. Stir.

Combine the mushrooms with the washed quinoa.

Pour in the white wine.

Pour in another cup of boiling water once most, but not all, of the water has evaporated.

Turn down the heat. This time, put a lid on the pot and simmer for an additional seven minutes.

Pour in an additional cup of boiling water.

Place a cover on it and simmer on low for 7 minutes.

This is what you ought to have after finishing.

Add some black pepper for seasoning. If more salt is needed, add it.

Incorporate manchego cheese and truffle oil.

Stir. There will be plenty of creamy risotto.

Add some chives as a garnish and serve right away.

BOOK 23:

Healthy snacks and sides

Healthy snacks and sides

Almond butter stuffed dates

Ingredients:

10 medjool dates

1/4 cup almond butter

1/4 cup chopped almonds (optional) A pinch of sea salt

Instructions:

Cut each date in half lengthwise and take out the pit.

Place around one spoonful of almond butter inside each date.

If preferred, top with chopped almonds and a little amount of sea salt. Serve right away or store in the fridge for up to a week.

Baked kale chips

Ingredients:

1 bunch kale, washed and dried 1 tablespoon olive oil

1/2 teaspoon sea salt

1/4 teaspoon garlic powder (optional)

Instructions:

Preheat the oven to 300°f or 150°c.

Remove the kale leaves from the stems and tear them into bite-sized pieces.

Add olive oil, sea salt, and garlic powder to the kale.

Spread out the kale in a single layer on a baking pan.

Bake for 10 to 15 minutes or until the edges are crispy but not browned.

After letting it cool, enjoy!

Carrot and hummus roll- ups

Ingredients:

2 large carrots, peeled and sliced into thin ribbons

1/2 cup hummus

Fresh parsley or cilantro for garnish

Instructions:

Arrange each carrot ribbon with a thin coating of hummus on it.

If necessary, secure the carrot ribbons with a toothpick after rolling them up. Add some cilantro or parsley as a garnish.

Serve right away or store in the fridge for up to a day.

Cauliflower buffalo wings

Ingredients:

1 small head cauliflower, cut into florets

1/2 cup flour 1/2 cup water

1 teaspoon garlic powder 1 teaspoon onion powder 1/2 teaspoon paprika 1/2 cup buffalo sauce

2 tablespoons melted butter or coconut oil

Instructions:

Turn the oven on to 450°f, or 230°c. Use parchment paper to line a baking sheet.

To make a batter, combine the flour, water, paprika, onion powder, and garlic powder in a bowl.

Place each cauliflower floret on the baking sheet after dipping it into the batter and brushing off any excess.

Bake, rotating halfway through, for 20 minutes.

Melt the butter or coconut oil and stir in the buffalo sauce.

After adding the buffalo sauce to the cooked cauliflower, toss it back in the oven for ten more minutes.

Accompany with your preferred dipping sauce.

Chia seed pudding with berries

Ingredients:

1/4 cup chia seeds

1 cup almond milk (or any milk of choice)

1 tablespoon maple syrup or honey 1/2 teaspoon vanilla extract

Fresh berries for topping

Instructions:

Combine the almond milk, vanilla extract, maple syrup, and chia seeds in a bowl.

Mix well to blend.

Stir once more to avoid clumping after letting it settle for five minutes.

For at least four hours or overnight, cover and chill.

Before serving, sprinkle fresh berries on top.

Cinnamon baked apples

Ingredients:

4 large apples, cored and sliced

1 tablespoon coconut oil or butter, melted

1 teaspoon cinnamon

1 tablespoon maple syrup or honey 1/4 cup chopped nuts (optional)

Instructions:

Set the oven's temperature to 175°c/350°f.

Combine cinnamon, melted butter or coconut oil, and honey or maple syrup with the apple slices.

Arrange the apples evenly on a baking dish.

If using, scatter some chopped nuts on top.

Bake the apples for 20 to 25 minutes or until they are soft.

Warm up and serve.

Coconut yogurt parfait

Ingredients:

1 cup coconut yogurt 1/2 cup granola

1/2 cup fresh berries

1 tablespoon honey or maple syrup

Instructions:

Arrange the granola, fresh berries, and coconut yogurt in a dish or glass.

Drizzle with maple syrup or honey. As desired, repeat the layers.

Serve right away.

Cucumber tomato salad with herbs

Ingredients:

2 cucumbers, sliced

1 pint cherry tomatoes, halved 1/4 red onion, thinly sliced 1/4 cup fresh parsley, chopped 1/4 cup fresh dill, chopped

2 tablespoons olive oil

1 tablespoon red wine vinegar Salt and pepper, to taste

Instructions:

Combine cucumbers, cherry tomatoes, red onion, parsley, and dill in a big bowl.

Mix the olive oil, red wine vinegar, salt, and pepper in a small bowl.

After adding the dressing to the salad, stir to mix. Serve right away or store in the fridge for up to a day.

Flaxseed and banana smoothie

Ingredients:

1 banana

1 tablespoon flaxseed meal

1 cup almond milk (or any milk of choice)

1/2 cup spinach (optional) 1/2 cup ice

1 teaspoon honey or maple syrup (optional)

Instructions:

Put everything into a blender. Blend till creamy and smooth. Serve right away.

Garlic roasted chickpeas

Ingredients:

1 can chickpeas, drained and rinsed 1 tablespoon olive oil

1 teaspoon garlic powder

1/2 teaspoon smoked paprika 1/2 teaspoon salt

Instructions:

Set oven temperature to 400°f, or 200°c.

Using a paper towel, pat the chickpeas dry.

Add salt, smoked paprika, garlic powder, and

olive oil to the chickpeas and toss.

Arrange the chickpeas in a single layer on a baking sheet.

Roast until crispy, stirring the pan halfway through, 20 to 30 minutes.

Before serving, allow it to cool somewhat.

BOOK 24:

Wholesome desserts

Wholesome desserts

Greek yogurt with honey and nuts

Ingredients:

200g Greek yogurt 2 tbsp honey

1/4 cup mixed nuts (almonds, walnuts, pistachios)

Instructions:

Spoon Greek yogurt into a bowl. Drizzle with honey.

Top with mixed nuts. Serve immediately.

Caprese skewers

Ingredients:

1 cup cherry tomatoes

1 cup fresh mozzarella balls Fresh basil leaves

Balsamic glaze

Instructions:

On small skewers, alternate cherry tomatoes, mozzarella balls, and basil leaves.

Arrange skewers on a platter.

Drizzle with balsamic glaze before serving.

Hummus and veggie sticks

Ingredients:

1 cup hummus

1 carrot, cut into sticks

1 cucumber, cut into sticks

1 red bell pepper, cut into sticks 1 celery stalk, cut into sticks

Instructions:

Arrange vegetable sticks on a platter. Serve with hummus for dipping.

Smoked salmon and cream cheese cucumber bites

Ingredients:

1 cucumber, sliced into rounds 100g smoked salmon

1/4 cup cream cheese Fresh dill for garnish

Instructions:

Spread a small amount of cream cheese on each cucumber round.

Top with a piece of smoked salmon. Garnish with fresh dill.

Turkey and cheese roll- ups

Ingredients:

100g sliced turkey breast

100g sliced cheese (cheddar, swiss, or your favorite)

Mustard or mayo (optional)

Instructions:

Lay a slice of turkey flat. Place a slice of cheese on top.

Spread a thin layer of mustard or mayo, if desired.

Roll up and secure with a toothpick. Repeat with remaining ingredients.

Chia seed coconut pudding

Ingredients:

1/4 cup chia seeds 1 cup coconut milk

1 tablespoon maple syrup or honey 1/2 teaspoon vanilla extract

Instructions:

Chia seeds, coconut milk, vanilla essence, and maple syrup or honey should all be combined in a bowl.

Mix well to blend.

Stir once more to avoid clumping after letting it settle for five minutes.

For at least four hours or overnight, cover and chill.

Accompany with raw fruit or a dash of grated coconut.

Cinnamon baked pears

Ingredients:

4 ripe pears, halved and cored

2 tablespoons maple syrup or honey 1 teaspoon cinnamon

1/4 teaspoon nutmeg

1/4 cup chopped nuts (optional)

Instructions:

Set the oven's temperature to 175°c/350°f.

The pear halves should be put in a baking dish.

Drizzle with honey or maple syrup. Add nutmeg and cinnamon on top.

If desired, garnish with chopped nuts. Bake the pears for 20 to 25 minutes or until they are soft.

Warm up and serve.

Date and nut bars

Ingredients:

1 cup dates, pitted and chopped

1 cup mixed nuts (almonds, walnuts, cashews)

1/4 cup shredded coconut 1 tablespoon chia seeds

1 tablespoon honey or maple syrup A pinch of sea salt

Instructions:

Put the dates, chia seeds, shredded coconut, mixed nuts, honey or maple syrup, and sea salt in a food processor. Process until a sticky dough develops and the ingredients comes together.

Line an 8 × 8-inch baking dish with parchment paper and press the mixture into it.

For minimum one hour, refrigerate. Slice into bars and keep chilled for a maximum of seven days.

Fig and walnut bites

Ingredients:

1 cup dried figs, stems removed 1/2 cup walnuts

1/4 cup rolled oats

1 tablespoon honey or maple syrup 1 teaspoon cinnamon

Instructions:

Blend the rolled oats, walnuts, honey, cinnamon, and dried figs in a food processor.

Process until the mixture forms a sticky dough and comes together.

Form dough into 1-inch spheres. Refrigerate the balls for a minimum of half an hour after placing them on a baking sheet covered with parchment paper.

For up to a week, keep in the refrigerator in an airtight container.

Transfer the blend into a low-profile container and place it in the freezer for

a minimum of 4 hours, stirring once per hour.

Before serving, let the sorbet soften for a few minutes at room temperature.

Ginger peach sorbet

Ingredients:

4 ripe peaches, peeled, pitted, and chopped

1/4 cup honey or maple syrup 1 tablespoon lemon juice

1 teaspoon fresh grated ginger

Instructions:

In a blender or food processor, add the diced peaches, honey (or maple syrup), lemon juice, and grated ginger. Process till smooth.

BOOK 25:

Whealing beverages and

Shopping Guides

Healing beverages

Chocolate-dipped strawberries

Ingredients:

200g fresh strawberries 100g dark chocolate

Instructions:

Melt dark chocolate in a microwave or double boiler. Dip each strawberry halfway into the melted chocolate. Place on a parchment-lined tray and let the chocolate set. Serve once the chocolate is firm.

Baked apples with cinnamon and nuts

Ingredients:

4 apples, cored

1/4 cup chopped walnuts 2 tbsp honey

1 tsp cinnamon

Instructions:

Preheat the oven to 180°c (350°f). Place cored apples in a baking dish. Fill the center of each apple with walnuts, honey, and cinnamon. Bake for 25-30 minutes, until apples are tender. Serve warm.

Greek yogurt parfait with berries

Ingredients:

200g Greek yogurt

1 cup mixed berries (blueberries, strawberries, raspberries)

2 tbsp honey 1/4 cup granola

Instructions:

In a glass, layer Greek yogurt, mixed berries, honey, and granola. Repeat the layers until the glass is full.

Serve immediately.

Chia seed pudding with fresh fruit

Ingredients:

1/4 cup chia seeds 1 cup almond milk 1 tbsp maple syrup

Fresh fruit (e.g., kiwi, mango, berries)

Instructions:

In a bowl, mix chia seeds, almond milk, and maple syrup. Stir well and refrigerate overnight.

In the morning, stir the pudding again and top with fresh fruit.

Avocado chocolate mousse

Ingredients:

2 ripe avocados

1/4 cup cocoa powder

1/4 cup honey or maple syrup 1 tsp vanilla extract

Pinch of salt

Instructions:

In a blender, combine avocados, cocoa powder, honey, vanilla extract, and salt. Blend until smooth and creamy.

Spoon the mousse into serving dishes and chill for at least 30 minutes before serving.

Coconut water electrolyte drink

Ingredients:

2 cups coconut water 1/2 cup orange juice 1/4 cup lemon juice

1 tablespoon honey or maple syrup A pinch of sea salt

Instructions:

Mix all the ingredients together in a pitcher.

To dissolve the honey or maple syrup, thoroughly stir. Refrigerate for a little before serving.

Detox green tea

Ingredients:

1 green tea bag

1 cup boiling water

1 tablespoon lemon juice

1 teaspoon honey or maple syrup A few fresh mint leaves (optional)

Instructions:

For three to five minutes, steep the green tea bag in hot water.

Take out the tea bag and mix in the honey or maple syrup and lemon juice. If desired, add some fresh mint leaves.
Serve warm or cold.

Energizing spirulina smoothie

Ingredients:

1 cup almond milk (or any milk of choice) 1 banana

1/2 cup frozen pineapple chunks 1 teaspoon spirulina powder

1 tablespoon chia seeds

1 tablespoon honey or maple syrup (optional)

Instructions:

Put everything into a blender. Blend till creamy and smooth. Serve right away.

Fennel digestive tea

Ingredients:

1 teaspoon fennel seeds

2 cups boiling water

Honey or lemon, to taste (optional)

Instructions:

Transfer the fennel seeds to an infuser or teapot. Cover the seeds with the boiling water.

Steep for five to ten minutes. Pour into cups after straining.

If desired, sweeten with honey or lemon.

Ginger lemonade golden milk

Ingredients:

2 cups milk (dairy or non-dairy)

1 teaspoon ground turmeric

1/2 teaspoon ground ginger

1 tablespoon honey or maple syrup

Instructions:

Heat Milk: In a saucepan set over medium heat, reheat the milk.

Include Spices: Add the turmeric and ground ginger and stir.

Add honey or maple syrup and stir until it dissolves to sweeten.

Simmer: For five minutes, lower the heat to a simmer.

To serve, transfer into mugs and consume warm.

I know from experience as a dietitian that many people find grocery shopping scary and daunting. For instance, a lot of my clients struggle to decide which foods to put in their basket at the grocery store and where to start.

Also, it can be challenging to distinguish between meals that are actually nutritious and those that are better left on the shelf due to the seemingly limitless options for food that are accessible, frequently in misleading packaging.

I walk you through the fundamentals of wise grocery shopping in this book, covering topics like making a well-thought-out shopping list, stocking up so you can shop less frequently, and selecting wholesome items.

Things to do Before you go shopping

Most people require some kind of plan, even if some individuals can shop for groceries without a list or a notion of the meals they'll prepare during the next week. If you tend to become distracted easily in the grocery store or are unsure of where to start, it would be a good idea to bring along a weekly menu or shopping list.

Creating a healthy shopping list

Many shoppers consider a grocery list to be an indispensable tool. It can assist you in staying focused and in remembering what you need. Also, research indicates that using a grocery list when shopping may encourage you to make healthier selections. However, what is in a "healthy" grocery shopping list?

In general, complete, nutrient-dense foods should make up the majority of a healthy, well-rounded diet. I refer to foods like fruits, vegetables, nuts, seeds, legumes, and sources of protein like fish and eggs. You should put these foods first on your list. Organizing your shopping list by categories, such as fruits, vegetables (starchy and nonstarchy), legumes and grains, nuts and seeds, proteins, frozen meals, dairy and nondairy alternatives, beverages, condiments, and other miscellaneous products, might be useful.

Planning a weekly menu

Alternatively, you can bring a weekly menu rather than a typical shopping list to the supermarket. The ingredients needed to prepare the meals you want to cook the week ahead of time can be found on this menu.

For instance, if you enjoy meal planning, try printing out the recipes you want to prepare. Next, just make purchases based on the ingredient listings.

Remember that making all of your meals and snacks at home might not be feasible if you're used to buying takeaway or eating out for most meals. For this reason, if you've never meal prepped before, start out small and aim to prepare a couple of meals in the first week.

You can expand your weekly culinary menu by adding extra meals once that becomes second nature. Just like with any healthy habit, it could take some time for you to get into the pattern of routinely going grocery shopping and cooking healthful meals at home.

How to read labels while shopping

Nothing in an item's packaging implies that it's unhealthy. Nevertheless, reviewing the nutrition information and ingredient labels of packaged goods is a good idea.

While highly processed, unhealthy meals typically have a lengthy ingredient list, some beneficial packaged foods also have this problem. Therefore, before deciding whether to buy something or leave it on the shelf, it's crucial to read the ingredient label.

I usually pass on something if the first few components are refined grains, highly processed oil or any kind of sugar.

The amount of added sugar in a food item is what I consider most important. Overindulging in added sugars can be detrimental to your general health and raise your risk of developing heart disease, mental health issues, and type 2 diabetes. For instance, I recently saw a readymade chai latte product at the grocery store. I was astonished to see that each 3/4-cup (180-mL) serving had an astounding 31 grams, or almost 8 teaspoons, of added sugar.

Although the packaging gave you the impression that it would be healthful by using terms like "organic" and "gluten-free," sugar syrup was the second component on the list.

Choosing products with less than 6 grams (1.5 teaspoons) of added sugar per serving is a smart idea when you're shopping for items like cereal or granola that typically contain some added sugar.

Weekly shopping lists

This is a weekly grocery list that follows a 30-day food plan. There are enough ingredients on this list to make all the meals that are scheduled for each week.

Week 1 shopping list

Proteins:

- Greek yogurt
- Chicken breasts
- Salmon fillets
- Shrimp
- Eggs
- Almond butter
- Mixed nuts
- Canned tuna
- Lentils

Fruits:

- Bananas
- Berries (strawberries, blueberries, mixed berries)
- Apples
- Oranges
- Lemons
- Avocados

- Pears

Vegetables:

- Mixed greens (spinach, kale)

- Cherry tomatoes

- Cucumbers

- Carrots

- Bell peppers

- Broccoli

- Sweet potatoes

- Asparagus Grains and legumes:

- Quinoa

- Brown rice

- Whole grain bread

- Whole grain pasta

- Whole grain crackers

- Oatmeal Dairy and alternatives:

- Almond milk (or any preferred milk)

- Cottage cheese Pantry

Staples:

- Olive oil

- Balsamic vinaigrette

- Honey

- Maple syrup

- Chia seeds

- Flaxseeds

- Protein powder

- Dark chocolate Herbs and spices:

- Fresh ginger

- Ground cinnamon

- Fresh mint

- Fresh parsley

- Ground turmeric

- Ground cumin

- Garlic

Beverages:

- Herbal tea (chamomile, green tea)

- Coconut water

Week 2 shopping list

Proteins:

- Chicken breasts

- Salmon fillets

- Ground beef

- Greek yogurt

- Eggs

- Almond butter

- Mixed nuts

- Canned tuna

- Lentils

- Black beans Fruits:

- Bananas

- Berries (strawberries, blueberries, mixed berries)

- Apples

- Oranges

- Avocados

- Lemons

- Pears

- Grapes

Vegetables:

- Mixed greens (spinach, kale)

- Cherry tomatoes

- Cucumbers

- Carrots

- Bell peppers

- Broccoli

- Sweet potatoes

- Asparagus

- Beets Grains and legumes:

- Quinoa

- Brown rice

- Whole grain bread

- Whole grain pasta

- Whole grain crackers

- Oatmeal Dairy and

Alternatives:

- Almond milk (or any preferred milk)

- Cottage cheese Pantry

Staples:

- Olive oil

- Balsamic vinaigrette

- Honey

- Maple syrup

- Chia seeds

- Flaxseeds

- Protein powder

- Dark chocolate Herbs and spices:

- Fresh ginger

- Ground cinnamon

- Fresh mint

- Fresh parsley

- Ground turmeric

- Ground cumin

- Garlic

Beverages:

- Herbal tea (chamomile, green tea)

- Coconut water

Week 3 shopping list

Proteins:

- Chicken breasts
- Salmon fillets
- Ground beef
- Greek yogurt
- Eggs
- Almond butter
- Mixed nuts
- Canned tuna
- Lentils
- Black beans Fruits:
- Bananas
- Berries (strawberries, blueberries, mixed berries)
- Apples
- Oranges
- Avocados
- Lemons
- Pears
- Grapes

Vegetables:

- Mixed greens (spinach, kale)
- Cherry tomatoes

- Cucumbers

- Carrots

- Bell peppers

- Broccoli

- Sweet potatoes

- Asparagus

- Beets Grains and

Legumes:

- Quinoa

- Brown rice

- Whole grain bread

- Whole grain pasta

- Whole grain crackers

- Oatmeal Dairy and

Alternatives:

- Almond milk (or any preferred milk)

- Cottage cheese Pantry

Staples:

- Olive oil

- Balsamic vinaigrette

- Honey

- Maple syrup

- Chia seeds

- Flaxseeds

- Protein powder

- Dark chocolate Herbs and spices:

- Fresh ginger

- Ground cinnamon

- Fresh mint

- Fresh parsley

- Ground turmeric

- Ground cumin

- Garlic

Beverages:

- Herbal tea (chamomile, green tea)

- Coconut water

Week 4 shopping list

Proteins:

- Chicken breasts

- Salmon fillets

- Ground beef

- Greek yogurt

- Eggs

- Almond butter

- Mixed nuts

- Canned tuna

- Lentils

- Black beans Fruits:

- Bananas

- Berries (strawberries, blueberries, mixed berries)

- Apples

- Oranges

- Avocados

- Lemons

- Pears

- Grapes

Vegetables:

- Mixed greens (spinach, kale)

- Cherry tomatoes

- Cucumbers

- Carrots

- Bell peppers

- Broccoli

- Sweet potatoes

- Asparagus

- Beets

Grains and legumes:

- Quinoa

- Brown rice

- Whole grain bread

- Whole grain pasta

- Whole grain crackers

- Oatmeal Dairy and

Alternatives:

- Almond milk (or any preferred milk)

- Cottage cheese Pantry

Staples:

- Olive oil

- Balsamic vinaigrette

- Honey

- Maple syrup

- Chia seeds

- Flaxseeds

- Protein powder

- Dark chocolate Herbs and spices:

- Fresh ginger

- Ground cinnamon

- Fresh mint

- Fresh parsley

- Ground turmeric

- Ground cumin

- Garlic

Beverages:

- Herbal tea (chamomile, green tea)

- Coconut water

30-day meal plan for optimal health.

Day 1: Balanced and nutritious

Breakfast: avocado toast on sprouted grain bread

Lunch: avocado quinoa salad with lemon dressing

Dinner: almond-crusted baked tofu

Day 2: Nutrient-dense and energizing

Breakfast: nutty banana smoothie

Lunch: black bean taco salad with cilantro-lime dressing

Dinner: barley and vegetable stew

Day 3: Refreshing and satisfying

Breakfast: berry spinach smoothie bowl

Lunch: cucumber noodle salad with peanut dressing

Dinner: butternut squash soup with sage

Snack: carrot and hummus roll-ups Dessert: mango lime chia pudding

Day 4: High energy day

Breakfast: sweet potato and black bean breakfast burritos

Lunch: sweet potato and kale buddha bowl

Dinner: broccoli almond stir-fry

Day 5: Relaxation and digestion

Breakfast: oatmeal with pumpkin seeds and pears

Lunch: broccoli and almond soup

Dinner: chickpea and spinach curry

Day 6: Detox focus

Breakfast: pineapple and kale smoothie

Lunch: curried cauliflower rice with cashews

Dinner: cauliflower steaks with herb sauce

Day 7: Heart health day

Breakfast: almond butter and banana oatmeal

Lunch: beetroot and spinach salad with walnuts

Dinner: eggplant lasagna with cashew ricotta

Day 8: Brain boosting day

Breakfast: spinach and avocado smoothie

Lunch: grilled portobello mushrooms with quinoa salad

Dinner: herbed mushroom and quinoa risotto

Day 9: Muscle maintenance day

Breakfast: quinoa breakfast bowl with almonds and berries

Lunch: lemon-garlic tempeh over brown rice

Dinner: lentil bolognese with zucchini noodles

Day 10: Sustainable energy day

Breakfast: chia seed pudding with kiwi

Lunch: mango and black bean quinoa bowl

Dinner: miso-glazed brussels sprouts

Day 11: Mental clarity day

Breakfast: overnight oats with almond butter and raspberry

Lunch: mixed greens with roasted pumpkin and pecans

Dinner: portobello mushroom fajitas

Day 12: Balanced mood day

Breakfast: spiced apple porridge

Lunch: cold lentil salad with sun-dried tomatoes

Dinner: pumpkin and chickpea tagine

Day 13: Gut health day

Breakfast: kale and mushroom tofu scramble

Lunch: roasted vegetables and farro bowl

Dinner: tomato basil spaghetti squash

Day 14: Immune boosting day

Breakfast: golden turmeric latte

Lunch: spiced chickpea stew with coconut milk

Dinner: pumpkin and chickpea tagine

Day 15: Healthy aging day

Breakfast: coconut yogurt parfait with mango

Lunch: spinach and strawberry salad with almonds

Dinner: roasted beet and walnut salad

Day 16: Stress reduction day

Breakfast: spinach and avocado smoothie

Lunch: lemon-garlic tempeh over brown rice

Dinner: herbed mushroom and quinoa risotto

Day 17: Metabolic boost day

Breakfast: pineapple and kale smoothie

Lunch: black bean taco salad with cilantro-lime dressing

Dinner: broccoli almond stir-fry

Day 18: Physical endurance day

Breakfast: nutty banana smoothie

Lunch: chickpea and avocado sandwich on sprouted bread

Dinner: sweet corn and black bean tacos

Day 19: Mental health focus day

Breakfast: berry spinach smoothie bowl

Lunch: baked sweet potato and hummus wrap

Dinner: spiced cauliflower and green beans

Day 20: Sleep enhancement day

Breakfast: chia seed pudding with kiwi

Lunch: cucumber noodle salad with peanut dressing

Dinner: cauliflower steaks with herb sauce

Day 21: Healthy skin day

Breakfast: coconut yogurt parfait with mango

Lunch: beetroot and spinach salad with walnuts

Dinner: pumpkin and chickpea tagine

Day 22: Immune support day

Breakfast: almond butter and banana oatmeal

Lunch: roasted vegetables and farro bowl

Dinner: miso-glazed brussels sprouts

Day 23: High fiber focus day

Breakfast: quinoa breakfast bowl with almonds and berries

Lunch: sweet potato and kale buddha bowl

Dinner: lentil bolognese with zucchini noodles

Day 24: Hormonal balance day

Breakfast: golden turmeric latte

Lunch: cold lentil salad with sun-dried tomatoes

Dinner: butternut squash soup with sage

Day 25: Athletic performance day

Breakfast: sweet potato and black bean breakfast burritos

Lunch: grilled portobello mushrooms with

quinoa salad

Dinner: sweet corn and black bean tacos

Day 26: Healthy aging day

Breakfast: coconut yogurt parfait with
mango

Lunch: spinach and strawberry salad with
almonds

Dinner: roasted beet and walnut salad

Day 27: Sleep enhancement
day

Breakfast: chia seed pudding with kiwi

Lunch: cucumber noodle salad with peanut
dressing

Dinner: cauliflower steaks with herb sauce

Day 28: Skin health day

Breakfast: coconut yogurt parfait with
mango

Lunch: beetroot and spinach salad with
walnuts

Dinner: pumpkin and chickpea tagine

Day 29: Cognitive function day

Breakfast: spinach and avocado smoothie

Lunch: lemon-garlic tempeh over brown rice

Dinner: herbed mushroom and quinoa risotto

Day 30: General wellness day

Breakfast: almond butter and banana oatmeal

Lunch: avocado quinoa salad with lemon
dressing

Dinner: almond-crusted baked tofu

Conclusion

I extend my heartfelt gratitude to all the readers who have chosen this book as their guide on the journey to better health and wellness. Your trust and interest are what inspire me to continue sharing knowledge and insights on natural healing and healthy living.

I also want to acknowledge the support of family and friends, whose encouragement and belief in the importance of this project have been unwavering. Your support has been a cornerstone in the creation of this encyclopedia.

Finally, I thank the editorial team for their hard work, meticulous attention to detail, and commitment to excellence. Your efforts have ensured that the information presented is accurate and accessible, making this book a reliable resource for all readers.

To you, my reader, I hope that this book serves as a valuable tool in your quest for health and well-being. Thank you for allowing me to be a part of your journey.

Printed in Great Britain
by Amazon

47017651R00231